# Handbook of Vestibular Rehabilitation

# Handbook of Vestibular Rehabilitation

### Edited by Linda M Luxon and
### Rosalyn A Davies

The National Hospital for Neurology and Neurosurgery,
London

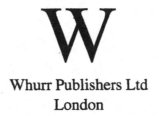

Whurr Publishers Ltd
London

© 1997 Whurr Publishers Ltd
First published 1997 by
Whurr Publishers Ltd
19b Compton Terrace, London N1 2UN, England

Reprinted 2000, 2001, 2002 and 2004

**British Library Cataloguing in Publication Data**
A catalogue record for this book is available from the British
Library

ISBN 1 86156 021 4

# Contents

# Contributors

From The National Hospital for Neurology and Neurosurgery, Queen Square, London WC1N 3BG

**Dr Rosalyn A Davies**
Consultant Physician in Neuro-otology

**Mr Alan Davidson**
Behavioural Nurse Therapist

**Mrs Gail Foord**
Senior Physiotherapist

**Dr Tina Laczko-Schroeder**
Senior Registrar in Department of Neuropsychiatry

**Professor Linda M Luxon**
Professor of Audiological Medicine, University College London and Consultant Physician in Neuro-otology

**Mrs Rachel Faber Rutley**
Senior Physiotherapist

**Dr Peter Savundra**
Senior Registrar in Audiological Medicine, Department of Neuro-otology

**Mr Steve Watson**
Audiological Scientist, Department of Neuro-otology

# Foreword

Luxon and Davies continue the rich clinical tradition in Neuro-otology at Queen Square in this outstanding Handbook of Vestibular Rehabilitation. They illustrate the importance of a team approach in dealing with the complex issues of vestibular rehabilitation. Since the time of Cawthorne and Cooksey, clinicians have been aware that vestibular compensation occurs more rapidly and is more complete if the patient begins exercising as soon as possible after a vestibular lesion. It has only been recently, however, that our understanding of vestibular adaptation and compensation have provided a physiologic underpinning for clinical observation. Controlled studies in animals have documented that exercise accelerates the compensation process after experimental vestibular lesions. A major strength of this handbook is that it provides the background in vestibular physiology and pathophysiology for understanding the key principles of vestibular rehabilitation.

This book will be valuable to anyone who provides clinical services for the dizzy patient. The multidisciplinary approach outlined by Luxon and Davies is unique in the field. I was particularly pleased to see that they included several chapters on psychological and behavioural therapies which are important but often neglected components in the management of the chronically dizzy patient. Since the authors have been working as a team, the handbook has a cohesive theme, a feature rarely achieved by such a multi-author text. The master list of references at the end of the text is another excellent feature that provides the reader with a concise list of the most up-to-date references in the field of vestibular rehabilitation. I have no doubt that this handbook will be invaluable for all clinicians, therapists, and paramedical staff involved in caring for the dizzy patient. There really is no other book that provides such a comprehensive yet cohesive approach to vestibular rehabilitation.

Robert W Baloh MD
Professor of Neurology,
UCLA School of Medicine,
Los Angeles, California.

# Preface

Two decades ago Sir Terence Cawthorne, Consultant Otolaryngologist to the National Hospital, collaborated with Dr Cooksey, a Rheumatologist at the King's College Hospital to develop the Cawthorne-Cooksey exercises for the management of dizziness after head injury. Their value in the management of all forms of peripheral vestibular disorder rapidly became apparent and formed the mainstay of treatment for this group of patients.

Over the last twenty years, this management strategy has been popularised and subsequent animal studies have shown the relevance of promoting visual, vestibular and proprioceptive inputs in a systematic and repetitive fashion to facilitate vestibular compensation.

This handbook is based on the lectures given at the first Vestibular Rehabilitation Training Day held at the National Hospital for Neurology and Neurosurgery, Queen Square, and is for clinicians, therapists and paramedical staff involved in the care of the dizzy patient. The programme was established in response to an increasing demand for clinical services for dizzy patients and a need to train both clinicians and other professionals in the methods of assessment and management of patients with disorientation. The strength of the rehabilitation programme at the National Hospital is based on the multidisciplinary approach and this is reflected by the contributions within this volume. The handbook aims to provide a practical overview of the relevant scientific background and clinical developments in the field of vestibular rehabilitation and outlines the strategy that has been developed at the National Hospital. It is the editors' hope that the contents of the book will provide not only a basic training manual, but will also promote the development of vestibular rehabilitation in a structured, effective and multidisciplinary way. Undoubtedly, the extension of vestibular rehabilitation programmes will raise questions, which, in time, will allow improvement and further developments in this field.

Linda M Luxon
Rosalyn A Davies

# Chapter 1
# The anatomy and physiology of vertigo and balance

PETER SAVUNDRA

## Introduction

This is an extremely complex topic but some understanding of vestibular anatomy and the psychophysiology of vertigo and balance is an essential prerequisite for those involved in the rehabilitation of patients with balance disorders (Savundra & Luxon, 1997).

This chapter will address only those aspects of anatomy and physiology which are of particular relevance to vestibular rehabilitation. For more detailed texts, readers are invited to consult appropriate sources (Baloh & Honrubia, 1990; Savundra & Luxon, 1997). The physiological basis of vestibular compensation is discussed in Chapter 2.

In humans, a highly sophisticated mechanism for maintaining gaze and balance has developed, which is dependent upon visual, vestibular, proprioceptive and superficial sensory information. This information is integrated in the central nervous system and is modulated by activity arising in the reticular formation, the extrapyramidal system, the cerebellum and the cerebral cortex. At every level from the vestibular receptors to the cerebral cortex, inputs are modulated by afferent and efferent pathways.

## Functions of the vestibular system

The vestibular system allows detection of body motion in all three planes, consequent upon linear and angular acceleration stimuli applied to the head. In addition, the vestibular system detects the gravitational vector, necessary for head and body orientations.

Vestibular information is integrated with other inputs to contribute to:

• The maintenance of the fovea on the object of visual fixation.

1

The vestibular system stabilises the fovea for high-frequency stimuli, such as occur during walking and running (>2 Hz) (Grossman et al., 1988), whereas the visual system stabilises the fovea for low-frequency stimuli. Without these stabilising systems, there would be a drop in visual acuity with head movements.

- Maintenance of balance.
- Activity of the autonomic nervous system.
- Level of arousal and mood.

## Symptomatology

A peripheral or central vestibular lesion may produce symptoms associated with a loss of balance, a failure of gaze fixation or an abnormality of perception. Although the vestibular system is important for balance, many patients can cope well with no vestibular function provided vision and proprioception remain intact. By contrast, a loss of proprioception can cause severe loss of balance.

Symptoms may be reported variously by patients as a specific illusion of movement or loss of balance to a much more vague complaint of dizziness, disequilibrium, faintness, giddiness, sensations of swimminess or floating, unexpected falls and anxiety or difficulty thinking in certain environments. The term *vertigo* is defined as the illusion of movement. The lay term *dizziness* can be used to cover the less-specific synonyms noted above. Other patients have an illusion of horizontal or vertical oscillation of the visual world, often precipitated by head movements, termed *oscillopsia*. Vertigo is often rotatory in nature even though the underlying eye movement abnormality may be horizontal in the form of *nystagmus*, repetitive eye movements with a slow and a fast component in opposite directions with no intervening time interval. The explanation for the perception of rotation is that during the slow eye movement, for example, to the left, the environment seems to move to the right over the retina, but during the fast phase there is no useful perception (Gresty, Trinder & Leech, 1976) before the next slow phase, during which the environment seems to continue to move to the right.

Sensory inputs are normally combined to provide an accurate model of the physical world, but symptoms arise when there is an unusual combination of sensory inputs triggered by exposure to visual stimuli, such as rapidly changing images on a television screen, striped material or fast-moving traffic and crowds. This is termed *visual vertigo*. Such symptoms can occur in the absence of demonstrable vestibular disease. From birth, the information required for balance is integrated and stored in data centres within different sites in the brain. New information is constantly compared with these data and under normal circumstances 'immediate recognition' of sensory patterns enables vestibular activity to occur at a subconscious level, but new data patterns, which are not immediately recognised, will precipitate the perception of vestibular activity.

The misleading sense of movement and disorientation may be associated with somatic symptoms, such as nausea and sweating and feelings of panic, anxiety and inadequacy. Similar symptoms have been described in space phobia and the importance of defining and differentiating a vestibular or visual disturbance is crucial in order to institute appropriate treatment.

## Anatomy and physiology

### Vestibular sensory epithelium

This is found in the three semicircular canals, utricle and saccule of each labyrinth. The sensory epithelium is localised to the maculae of the utricle and saccule and the cristae ampullares of the semicircular canals. The sensory cells (vide infra) are surrounded by supporting cells, and therefore do not come into direct contact with the bony base of the cristae. The apical surfaces of the supporting cells are covered with microvilli. Close to the periphery of the sensory epithelium of the utricular macula and the cristae are the dark cell regions (Kimura, 1969). These cells resemble those of the stria vascularis and are thought to secrete vestibular endolymph and contribute to its electrical potential. Uniquely, endolymph has a positive potential, the stability of which is essential for vestibular function.

### Macula

Each macula is a small area of sensory epithelium. The ciliary bundles of the sensory cells project into the overlying statoconial membrane, which consists of an otoconial layer, a gelatinous area and a subcupular meshwork. The otoconial layer comprises calcareous material: the gelatinous layer, a mucopolysacchride gel, and the subcupular layer, a honeycomb of ciliary bundles. The otoconia are of variable size, but are distributed in a characteristic pattern. In the saccule, the largest otoconia are found close to the central strip (the striola) of the saccule, whereas in the utricle it is the smallest that lie near the striola, with the largest nearer the periphery of the macula. The sensory cells are also organised with the kinocilia orientated away from the striola in the saccular macula, but towards the striola in the utricular macula. This orientation is of considerable importance in understanding the physiology of the saccule and the utricle (vide infra). The otoconia appear to have a slow turnover. They are produced by the supporting cells of the sensory epithelium (Harada, 1979) and are resorbed by the dark cell regions (Lim, 1984).

The specific gravity of the otoconial membrane is approximately 2.7. Therefore, even at rest, it exerts a force on the sensory epithelium.

### Crista

The semicircular canals each consist of an endolymph-filled canal with a dilated area, the ampulla, in which lies the cupula, which rests on the crista. The crista ampullaris consists of a crest of sensory epithelium supported on a mound of connective tissue, laying at right angles to the longitudinal axis of the canal. The crista is surmounted by a bulbous, wedge-shaped, gelatinous mass, the cupula. The cilia of the sensory cells project into the cupula. The exact anatomy of the cupula *in vivo* is uncertain as preparation is associated with its shrinkage and the effect of this on its structure is unknown. *In vivo*, it may form a watertight seal, acting as a swing-door (Steinhausen, 1931) or a modified elastic diaphragm (McLaren & Hillman, 1979) with endolymph movement, or there might be a small, subcupular space, through which endolymph can pass (Dohlman, 1938). With either model the stereocilia would be deflected with head movements or change in the gravitational vector.

The specific gravity of the cupula is the same as that of endolymph, although, because of its different composition it may have different solubility coefficients for different solutes, for example, ethanol. This could lead to differences in specific gravity under different conditions and explain, for example, vertigo after alcohol and the 'morning after' effect. At rest, under normal conditions, the cupula does not exert a force on the sensory epithelium.

### Vestibular receptor cells

There are a total of 23 000 hair cells in the three human cristae and about 40 000 in the two maculae (Figure 1.1). The hair cells are surrounded by supporting cells, which are attached to the basement membrane, in which is found the neural and neurovascular tissue. The sensory cells are neuroepithelial hair cells, each bearing 50–100 thin stereocilia and a single thick and long kinocilium on the apical surface (Kikuchi et al., 1989). The stereocilia, which are non-motile and rigid, are not true cilia, but consist of actin filaments in a paracrystalline array, and other cytoskeletal proteins (Flock & Cheung, 1977). The stereocilia vary in height, but are graded with reference to the kinocilium, the tallest — about 100 $\mu$m — being closest to the kinocilium. There are crosslinks between the stereocilia and the kinocilium.

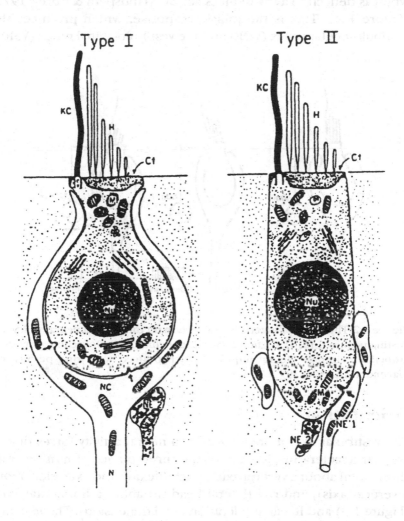

**Figure 1.1** The two types of vestibular hair cells. kC = kinocilium; H = hairs; Ct = cuticular plate; M = mitochondria; Nu = nucleus; NC = afferent nerve chalice; NE1 = afferent nerve bouton; NE2 = efferent nerve bouton.

There are at least two types of vestibular hair cell, which differ in morphology, function and innervation (Wersall & Bagger-Sjoback, 1974).

At rest, there is a continuous discharge from the afferent nerves of the hair cells (Fernandez & Goldberg, 1971, 1976). This is the tonic output, which in health is balanced by the tonic output from the contralateral labyrinth. Any asymmetry would cause a tendency for deviation of the eyes, leading to nystagmus, postural changes causing instability and the perception of vertigo. The deflection of the stereocilia towards the kinocilium increases afferent activity, whereas deflection away reduces activity (Hudspeth & Corey, 1977) (Figure 1.2). This is the phasic response, which produces the vestibulo-ocular reflex (VOR) and the vestibulo-spinal reflex (VSR).

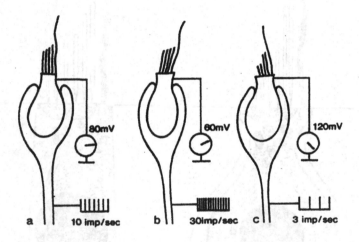

**Figure 1.2** The effect of stereociliar deflection on the afferent neural volley. (a) Resting position; (b) Deflection towards kinocilium; (c) Deflection away from kinocilium. imp = Neural impulses. (Reproduced with kind permission (Savundra & Luxon, 1997).)

## Orientation

The vestibular system transduces into neural activity forces due to angular acceleration in each of the three planes of motion: yaw (horizontal about a vertical axis); pitch (flexion and extension about a vertical axis), and roll (lateral head tilt about a horizontal axis) (Figure 1.3) and linear acceleration in all dimensions. The maximal stimulus is a force parallel to the surface of the sensory epithelium (Békésy, 1966), whereas a force perpendicular to the surface is ineffective (Fernandez & Goldberg, 1976).

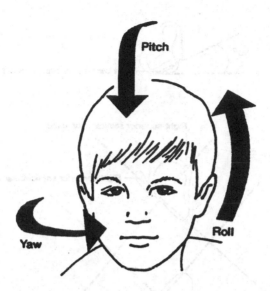

**Figure 1.3** The three planes of head movement. (Reproduced with kind permission (Savundra & Luxon, 1997).)

The anatomical organisation of the components of the vestibular system contribute to the analysis of these stimuli (Figure 1.4). The labyrinths are sited on the horizontal axis of the cranium. The lateral semicircular canals slope downwards and backwards at an angle of approximately 30° to the horizontal. The two vertical canals are approximately orthogonal to one another. The superior vertical canal is anterior and is directed postero-medially to antero-laterally over the roof of the utricle. The posterior vertical canal is posterior and is directed downward and laterally behind the utricle. The ipsilateral posterior and contralateral superior canals are approximately in the same plane, although precise measurements indicate that the canals are not in perfect geometric alignment.

The sensory epithelium is also spatially arranged. The cristae lie at right angles to the longitudinal axis of the canals and are, therefore, in the optimal plane for stimulation following displacement of the cupula or endolymph. Both maculae lie along the contours of the labyrinth: the utricular macula approximately in the horizontal plane and the saccula macula, on the medial wall, in approximately the vertical plane. The contours of the saccule and utricle further enhance the complexity of the orientation of their sensory epithelium.

The hair cells are also spatially orientated. In the maculae, the hair cells are orientated with reference to the S-shaped striolae (Figure 1.5). In the saccular macula, the kinocilia are orientated

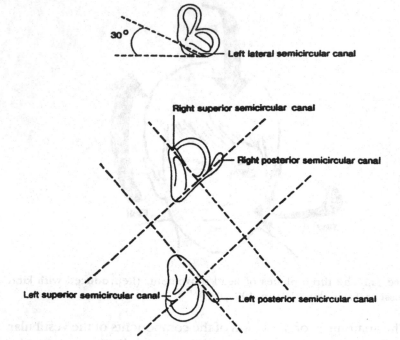

Figure 1.4 The orientation of the semicircular canals. (Reproduced with kind permission (Savundra & Luxon, 1997).)

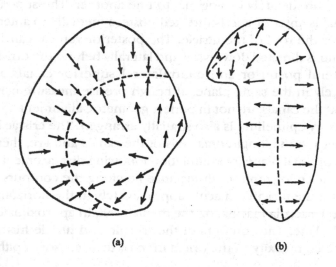

Figure 1.5 Orientation of hair cells of (a) utricular and (b) saccular maculae with reference to the striolae. (Arrow head indicates direction of kinocilia; broken line = striola.)

away from the striola, while in the utricular macula, the kinocilia are orientated towards the striola. Therefore, subtle differences in the displacement of the otoconial membrane will produce different patterns of responses from the hair cells. However, the orientation of the utricular macula is likely to make it more sensitive to horizontal (side to side) linear acceleration, whereas that of the saccular macula is likely to make it more sensitive to vertical (head–toe) linear acceleration.

The orientation of the hair cells of the lateral semicircular canals makes them most sensitive to yaw movements. The vertical canals are more sensitive to pitch and roll, with the posterior semicircular canal most response to pitch with the head in the yaw position (i.e. with the jaw approximated to the shoulder).

The three-dimensional orientation of the vestibular system is of clinical significance:

* The Hallpike manoeuvre specifically stimulates the posterior semicircular canal.
* Rotation about a vertical axis stimulates both lateral canals simultaneously.
* The head tilted is 30° down in rotation testing to maximise lateral canal stimulation.
  The patient lies at 30° to place the lateral canal vertical in the caloric test.
* Patients with vertigo who walk looking down will increase the stimulation of the lateral canals perhaps highlighting a canal asymmetry.
* It is difficult to test the anterior semicircular canals and the utricle and saccule.

# Central modulation

The result of head rotation in the yaw plane is to stimulate the ipsihorizontal canal and inhibit the horizontal canal. The effect is further enhanced by the neuronal pattern of excitation and inhibition. The ipsilateral canal stimulates the ipsilateral bipolar primary afferent neurons, whose cell bodies lie in Scarpa's ganglion (Fernandez & Goldberg, 1971; Fuchs & Kimm, 1975). These excite Type I secondary vestibular neurons in the vestibular nuclei which, in turn, excite contralateral Type II neurons, which inhibit the contralateral Type I neurons (Shimazu & Precht, 1966; Markham, Yagi & Curthoys, 1977). Further inhibition of the contralateral Type I neurons is effected by another inhibitory pathway from the reticular substance. Type I neurons are also excited by the ipsilateral fastigial nucleus, which is under the inhibitory influence of the cerebellar Purkinje cells. Type II neurons are excited by the contralateral fastigial nucleus and also by commissural fibres (Pompeiano, 1974; Highstein et al., 1987). It is likely that this central modulation has an important time domain function and may explain the phenomenon of central velocity storage, the time constant of the VOR considerably exceeding the time constant of cupular deflection (Raphan, Matsuo & Cohen, 1979). The vestibular nuclei also receive a pathway from the visual system.

## Ascending and descending vestibular projections

The vestibular nuclei have projections to the reticular formation, the cerebellum, the contralateral vestibular nuclei, the III, IV and VI cranial nuclei, the vestibulospinal tracts, the autonomic nervous system and thalamo-cortical projections, including the inferior parietal sulcus, anterior cingulate gyrus and primary sensory cortex (Bottini et al., 1994) (Figure 1.6). There are also descending projections to the vestibular nuclei from the cerebellum and reticular formation (Highstein, 1991). There are efferent projections to the vestibular sensory epithelium from an area near the vestibular nuclei and the sensitivity of the vestibule is under efferent control with the involvement of several transmitters, including calcitonin-gene related peptide (Tanaka et al., 1989), substance P (Usami, Hozawi & Ylikoski, 1991), acetylcholine and GABA (Lopez & Meza, 1988). There is also a large autonomic output to the labyrinth, the function of which is unknown.

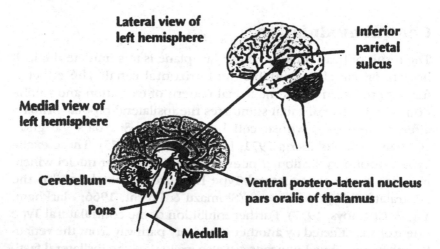

**Figure 1.6** The ascending vestibular projections.

The perception and responses to vestibular stimulation and pathology are therefore complex and are not predictable on the basis of the stimulus parameters.

## Arterial supply

The labyrinth, vestibulo-cochlear nerve and facial nerve are supplied by an end artery, the *labyrinthine* or *internal auditory* artery, but there may be one (30%), two (54%), three (14%) or four (2%) such arteries in a cerebellopontine angle. These two cranial nerves also receive branches from the *recurrent perforating branches* of the *anterior inferior cerebellar artery*. The *labyrinthine arteries* are branches of the *anterior inferior cerebellar artery*, which also supplies the pons and cerebellum. The *labyrinthine arteries* have two main branches: the *common cochlear artery* and the *anterior vestibular artery*. The former divides in the internal auditory canal into the *vestibulocochlear artery* and the *spiral modiolar artery* (cochlear artery). The *vestibulocochlear artery* divides into the *posterior vestibular artery* and the *cochlear branch*. The *anterior vestibular artery* supplies the utricle, a portion of the saccule and the anterior and lateral semicircular canals. The *posterior vestibular artery* supplies the major part of the saccule, the posterior semicircular canal and the lower part of the basal turn of the cochlea while the *cochlear branch* runs in the opposite direction towards the apex. The *spiral modiolar artery* enters the modiolus about half a turn from the basal end of the cochlea and runs towards the apex giving off the *external* and *internal radiating arterioles*. There are anastomoses between the *cochlear branch* and the *spiral modiolar artery* (Figure 1.7).

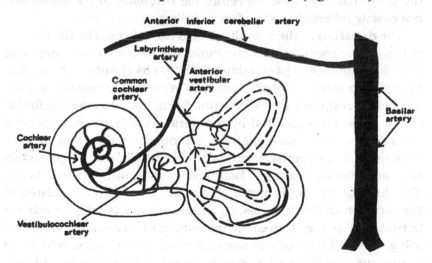

**Figure 1.7** The labyrinthine arterial circulation. (After Axelsson, 1974.)

Vertebrobasilar insufficiency is frequently considered part of the differential diagnosis in patients with vertigo due to change of head position and is often considered a contraindication to vestibular rehabilitation exercises, but it should be noted that the arteries, which supply the central and peripheral vestibular structures, also supply other areas of the pons and medulla and it would be expected that the patient would develop symptoms and signs indicative of ischaemia to adjacent areas and not only vertigo if the true diagnosis were vertebrobasilar insufficiency.

## The effect of head movements

Due to the inertia of the endolymph of the semicircular canals and the otoconia of the utricular and saccular maculae, a head movement will cause deflection of the cupula and stereocilia of the vestibular hair cells. This leads to an increase or decrease in the tonic output of the primary afferent neurons dependent on whether the stereocilia were deflected towards or away from the kinocilia. The afferent neurons have an asymmetric response with a greater increase than decrease in firing rate (Fernandez & Goldberg, 1976). Therefore, the pattern of the afferent neural discharge gives information on the **direction** of the stimulus in comparison with the gravitational vector. For small movements, the magnitude of cupula deflection is proportional to cranial velocity and this is reflected by the primary afferent neural response, but this does not match head velocity exactly, with a phase lead at high frequencies and adaptation at low frequencies (Melville Jones, 1974). In addition, there is an efferent output, which modulates the response of the vestibular hair cells. Therefore the **intensity** of the stimulus is not exactly reflected by the afferent volley.

The **duration** of the stimulus is also not reflected by the afferent volley. A few seconds after the cupula is deflected by a step-wise stimulus, cupula mechanics determine that its elasticity returns it to its resting position (Melville Jones, 1974) with a return of the afferent neural response to the baseline firing rate, but the vestibular-ocular response, measured by the duration of nystagmus, persists 5–10 times as long and it has been demonstrated that even after the cessation of nystagmus, there is an after-effect due to persisting vestibular nuclei activation lasting several minutes (Hood, 1973). The duration of the response, therefore, is not directly related to the duration of the stimulus. In addition, there is little correlation between the **perception** of the magnitude of acceleration and physiological variables, such as the duration, amplitude or velocity of nystagmus (van Egmond, Groen & Jongkees, 1948; Guedry, 1974).

# Vestibular responses

There are three types of response following peripheral vestibular stimulation: the VOR, VSR and the vestibulo-collic reflex (VCR) (Table 1.1).

**Table 1.1** Vestibular responses

---

- Vestibulo-ocular
    - semicircular canal-ocular response
    - otolith-ocular response
- Vestibulo-spinal
- Vestibulo-collic

---

VORs include the semicircular canal-ocular reflexes and the otolith-ocular reflexes.

## Semicircular canal-ocular reflexes

This is the dominant VOR and the measurement of the lateral semicircular canal-ocular reflexes, by examination of the oculomotor responses to precise vestibular stimuli, is of immense clinical value.

An angular acceleration to the right in the plane of the lateral canals would cause endolymph displacement to the left, leading to utriculopetal deviation of the cupula of the right lateral canal with utriculofugal movement of the cupula of the left lateral canal (Figure 1.8). This results in an increase in the firing rate of the right ampullary nerve, with a decrease in neural activity in the left ampullary nerve, and a subsequent contraction of the left lateral rectus and the right medial rectus muscles, with relaxation of the left medial rectus and the right lateral rectus muscles, producing deviation of the eyes to the left (Cohen, Suzuki & Bender, 1964).

## Vestibulo-spinal reflexes (VSR)

The labyrinth influences posture and orientation through neck, axial and limb motorneurons. However, the influence of vestibular activity on postural muscles is more difficult to define and less clearly understood than the labyrinthine control of eye movements (Anderson, Soechting & Terzuolo, 1979).

Alterations in vestibular function can profoundly affect posture (Figure 1.9). Ewald (1892) demonstrated such changes in posture by rotating animals on a turntable; when rotation ceased, the animal showed a tendency to fall in the direction of the slow phase

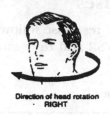

Direction of head rotation
RIGHT

Vestibulo-ocular reflex
SLOW PHASE OF NYSTAGMUS TO LEFT

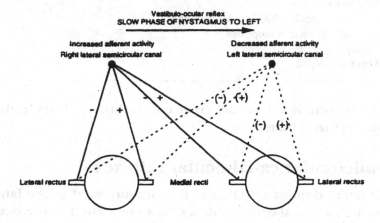

**Figure 1.8** The vestibulo-ocular reflex (VOR). – = Inhibition; + = Excitation; (+) = Disinhibition (reduced inhibition); (–) = Disfacilitation (reduced excitation). (Reproduced with kind permission (Savundra & Luxon, 1997).)

of eye movement and head deviation. This tendency was counteracted by a reflex increase in extensor tone in the antigravity muscles of the limb, on the side towards which the animal was falling, with a simultaneous reduction of extensor tone in the contralateral limbs. The animal, therefore, maintained its balance. These reflexes are mediated by a push–pull mechanism between the extensor and flexor muscles.

The vestibular apparatus exerts an influence on the control of posture by way of the myotatic reflex (the deep tendon reflex). Impulses are transmitted to alpha- and gamma-motoneurons of the spinal cord and body posture is maintained through the maculo-spinal reflex arc. This reflex is under the influence not only of the vestibular system but also of the multiple supraspinal centres, including the basal ganglia, the cerebellum and the reticular formation. The vestibular influence may be demonstrated in animals by the ipsilateral reduction of muscular tone, following unilateral destruction of the labyrinth or the lateral vestibular nucleus.

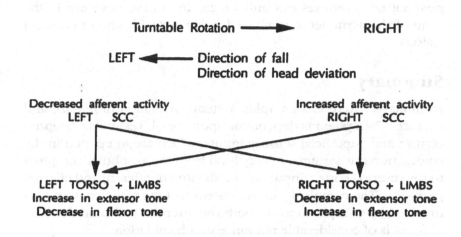

Figure 1.9 The reciprocal arrangement of the canal-spinal reflex (VSR). SCC = Semicircular canal. (Reproduced with kind permission. (Savundra & Luxon, 1997).)

## Proprioception and the cervico-ocular reflex

Proprioception has the major role in balance. A loss of lower limb proprioception or a cortical sensory loss severely compromises balance. The multisensory dizziness syndrome of Drachman and Hart (1972) is due to mixed visual, vestibular and proprioceptive loss together with associated musculoskeletal pathology.

Cervical proprioception is a function of the deep short muscles of the neck, which are rich in muscle spindles (Richmond & Bakker, 1982). Proprioception is also mediated by the Pacini receptors and Golgi tendon organs of periarticular tissue (McCloskey, 1978). If the cervical apophyscal joints are infiltrated with local anaesthetic, the subject can feel vertiginous and will tend to fall towards the side of the injection (de Jong et al., 1977) and unilateral electrical stimulation of the neck or trunk tilt with the head fixed can cause deviation of the subjective vertical. The role of cervical proprioception in maintaining ocular stability is uncertain. Horizontal contralateral nystagmus has been reported with cervical anaesthesia (de Jong et al., 1977). Cutaneous and limb proprioception also have an uncertain role, but nystagmus can be evoked in stationary subjects seated in darkness inside a rotating cylinder by placing their hands on the inner wall (Brandt, Buchele & Arnold, 1977).

Cervical proprioception mediates two reflexes: the cervico-ocular reflex and tonic postural neck reflexes. In humans, tonic postural neck reflexes can only be elicited in the newborn in the form of the asymmetric tonic neck reflex, or with gross brainstem lesions.

## Summary

In humans, there is a complex system for maintaining gaze and balance. The system is dependent upon visual, vestibular, proprioceptive and superficial sensory inputs, which are integrated in the central nervous system. At every level from the vestibular receptors to the cerebral cortex, inputs are modulated by afferent and efferent pathways. The complexity of the system and the many components involved have implications in both the intensity and time domains and this is of considerable relevance to rehabilitation.

The particular three-dimensional orientation of the vestibular system offers exquisite directional sensitivity, but there is little correlation between other stimulus parameters and the perception of their magnitude, particularly for small head movements, and this clearly has implications for the rehabilitation of patients with vertigo due to vestibular pathology.

Although the vestibular system is important for balance, many patients cope well with no vestibular function. Similarly vision is important for balance, but eye closure does not cause balance problems in the otherwise unimpaired and the blind have good balance. By contrast, a loss of proprioception can cause a severe loss of balance. This has implications for the rehabilitation of balance in patients with vestibular pathology.

There is considerable interaction between the vestibular system and the reticular formation and the limbic system, and vestibular inputs influence levels of arousal and mood and autonomic responses. Therefore consideration should be given to a holistic approach in the management of patients with vestibular disorders and a purely mechanistic approach is likely to be unsuccessful in many cases.

# Chapter 2
# Vestibular compensation

LINDA M LUXON

A plethora of different pathological processes (see Chapter 3) may affect the peripheral vestibular apparatus and give rise to a variety of different clinical syndromes, depending on the severity, extent and involvement of the five different vestibular receptor organs within the labyrinth. The presenting clinical syndromes vary from acute vertigo, associated with nausea and vomiting, characteristic of acute labyrinthitis, to the more varied and insidious presentations of patients reporting bizarre symptoms, such as 'they feel as though they are in a goldfish bowl watching their life go by' or they feel 'their brain is slopping around inside their skull'. While loss of hair cells within a vestibular sensory receptor will not recover (vestibular regeneration has not been documented in Man), in most cases the associated symptoms gradually abate and the patient becomes asymptomatic, usually over a period of 3–4 weeks to several months. The processes, which bring about the resolution of vestibular symptoms are collectively known as cerebral compensation and are usually attributed to cerebral plasticity, in which sensory inputs, somatosensory afferents and remaining labyrinthine function facilitate changes in the central nervous system and rapid reorganisation of vestibular circuits allowing recovery of symptomatology. Functional recovery depends on the restoration of perfect balance by reduction or abolition of the asymmetry in postural and oculomotor tone and recalibration of the gain of the dynamic vestibular reflexes, in order to ensure symmetrical compensatory vestibulo-spinal and vestibulo-ocular reflex (VOR) action, during movements of the head and body.

The causes of failure of compensation or intermittent decompensation are not clear, but cerebellar damage, impairment of proprioception, visual impairment and psychological disorders, with intercurrent physical illness have all been cited as possible contributing factors (Rudge & Chambers, 1982).

17

In rehabilitation terms, the failure of compensation for a vestibular impairment, which is defined as deranged function, may lead to a disability, i.e. a problem with balance arising directly from the impairment (Table 2.1). This, in turn, may lead to a handicap, which refers to the general effects on the individual's life, arising indirectly from the vestibular dysfunction.

**Table 2.1** Definitions of impairment, disability and handicap (WHO, 1980)

| | |
|---|---|
| Impairment | implies deranged function |
| Disability | refers to the balance problems as a result of the impairment |
| Handicap | refers to the general effects on the individual's life arising indirectly from the vestibular dysfunction |

This downward spiral is represented in Figure 2.1, in which a unilateral labyrinthine dysfunction leads to the disability of veering to one side while walking and thus to the handicap of a fear of going out and isolation. Thus, in rehabilitation terms compensation for a labyrinthine impairment is vital in rendering the patient asymptomatic, and preventing, or reducing, the development of disability and handicap (WHO, 1980).

## WHO schema for disablements

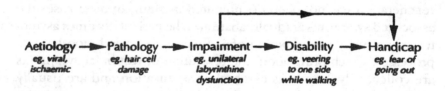

Aetiology → Pathology → Impairment → Disability → Handicap
eg. viral, ischaemic / eg. hair cell damage / eg. unilateral labyrinthine dysfunction / eg. veering to one side while walking / eg. fear of going out

**Figure 2.1** The relationship of impairment to disability and handicap in vestibular pathology.

# Pathophysiology

In the normal situation (Figure 2.2), vision, proprioception and vestibular inputs combine to provide an accurate model of the physical world, but symptoms of dysequilibrium may develop when there is an unusual combination of sensory inputs. Physiologically, this may occur in response to unusual visual stimuli, such as rapidly moving visual targets (for example, on a television screen, or on a full-field circularama theatre). This phenomenon has been explained on the basis that the information required for balance is integrated and modulated within the central nervous system in a 'database', with which all new information related to balance is constantly compared. In all familiar and normal situations, the information is immediately 'recognised' and subconscious vestibular activity occurs, but when unrecognised and unusual data are presented, this 'mismatch' becomes consciously perceived and is accompanied by a sense of disorientation and motion (Roberts, 1978).

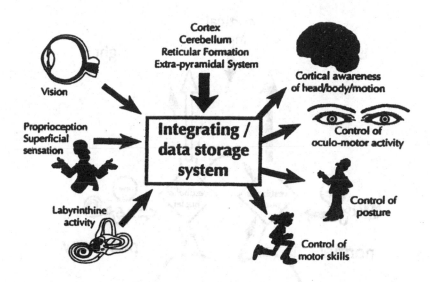

**Figure 2.2** The normal mechanisms subserving balance. (From Savundra & Luxon, 1997, reproduced with permission.)

Pathologically, the perception of motion of self and/or of the environment may be provoked by vestibular, visual or neurological disease, as the sensory inputs in the pathological state no longer 'match' the 'expected' and recognised inputs for any given stimulus. In the motorist's disorientation syndrome, Page and Gresty (1985) identified patients with vestibular disease, who developed an illusion of excessive turning and made inappropriate steering adjustments, when turning at speed. The unexpected and misleading sense of motion may be associated with somatic symptoms, such as nausea, sweating, panic, anxiety and fear.

Electrophysiological studies indicate that following labyrinthectomy, there is a loss of activity in the ipsilateral, secondary, vestibular neurones of the vestibular nuclei. Subsequently, however, there is a return of activity to the deafferented vestibular neurones on the damaged side, suggesting that these neurones recover spontaneous activity (Precht, Shimazu & Markham, 1966), which serves to redress the imbalance of vestibular neural activity within the whole vestibular system. The initial loss of ipsilateral activity is accompanied by a reduction of activity in the vestibular neurones of the contralateral nuclei, which also helps to reduce the marked neural asymmetry generated within the vestibular apparatus and is thought to be mediated by cerebellar inhibition of the contralateral vestibular nuclei (Figure 2.3).

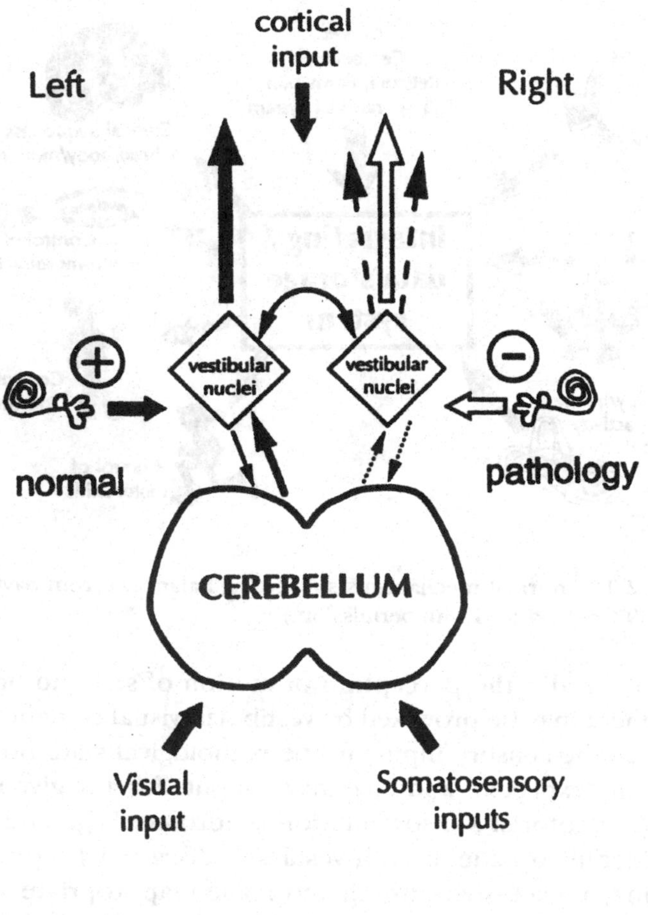


**Figure 2.3** The pathophysiological mechanisms subserving vestibular compensation (⊖= reduced activity; ⊕ = normal activity; ⇨= impaired activity; ⇢= reduced activity between vestibular nuclei on damaged side and cerebellum; ⇆ = increased inhibition between cerebellum and vestibular nuclei on 'normal' side; ⟶= spontaneous recurrence of neural activity from vestibular nuclei on damaged side.)

Recovery and rehabilitation of the vestibulo-ocular and vestibulo-spinal reflexes have been reported to be more rapid after labyrinthectomy than after vestibular nerve section, suggesting that the vestibular nerve contributes in some way to compensation (Cass & Goshgarian, 1991). These functions do not recover so effectively, if the lesion involves the central vestibular connections (Petrone, de Benedittis & de Candia, 1991).

The structures subserving compensation for vestibular dysfunction are unknown, but it has been shown that brainstem, cerebellar and cortical structures are involved, in addition to the requirement for all sensory inputs, including vision, somatosensory afferents and remaining labyrinthine input, which are involved in the perception of space, body posture and body locomotion (Lacour & Xerri, 1984).

There is considerable evidence for the involvement of the cerebellum in the modulation of vestibular activity, particularly the interaction of visual and vestibular information (Ito, 1972). The cerebellum receives not only vestibular information from first and second order vestibular neurones but also visual input via climbing fibres from the dorsal cap of the inferior olive, which pass on to the Purkinje cells of the cerebellar flocculus. Haddad, Demer and Robinson (1980) have demonstrated that ablation of the dorsal cap of the inferior olive compromises the plasticity of the vestibular system. In terms of the documented electrophysiological findings noted above, it has been shown that, whereas cerebellectomy, spinal cord section and mid-line mid-brain section do not reduce the recovery of spontaneous activity in the vestibular nuclei, the cerebellum and the commissural fibres act to reduce the activity of the contralateral vestibular nuclei. Thus, it would seem likely that the compensatory processes may involve these pathways (McCabe, Ryu & Sekitani, 1972; Schaefer & Meyer, 1973). The cerebellum, therefore, is a key centre for integration of different sensory information and, if intact, a relatively rapid reorganisation of vestibular circuits can be achieved following vestibular pathology.

The physiological mechanisms subserved by these various anatomical substrates required for compensation also remain poorly defined. Lacour, Roll and Appaix (1976) demonstrated that restraining a baboon in a plaster cast inhibited compensation (Figure 2.4), whereas Igarashi and coworkers (1981) demonstrated that 2½ hours' daily exercise improved gait deviation in unilateral labyrinthectomised squirrel monkeys. Similarly, Courjon et al. (1977) demonstrated that visual input allowed a more rapid loss of spontaneous nystagmus than captivity in the dark, after hemi-labyrinthectomy in the cat. Moreover, Fetter, Zee and Proctor (1988) have shown that occipital lobectomy, prior to labyrinthectomy, results in impaired compensation and recovery, while Schaefer and Meyer (1973) have demonstrated that cervical transection leading to a loss of proprioception also delays vestibular compensation.

The most widely accepted hypothesis to explain these observations is that of *central nervous system plasticity*, which refers to the ability of the central nervous system to adapt to altered sensory input and maintain an appropriate response. As noted above, the cerebellum is deemed to be extremely important in this function and the vestibular system has been shown to be extremely adaptable. Prisms may cause the visual perception of moving targets to be reversed and yet normal subjects can learn to compensate and function well. This compensation extends as far as the reversal of the VOR following rotation in the dark (Gonshore & Melvill Jones, 1976).

In animals, vestibular compensation may in part be explained on the basis of reactive synaptogenesis, with the development of new synapses and axonal sprouts. Although this has been documented in the frog (Dieringer, Kunzle & Precht, 1984), it has not been demonstrated in mammals. Following denervation, supersensitivity to neurotransmitters may also develop, although this has not been

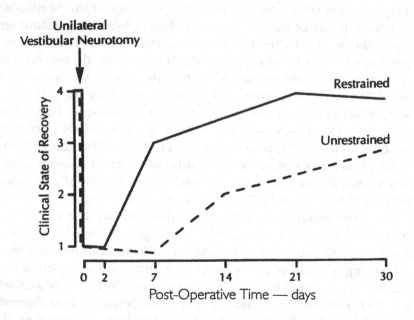

**Figure 2.4** Functional balance recovery in restrained and unrestrained baboons following unilateral vestibular neurotomy. (After Lacour, Roll & Appaix, 1976.)

demonstrated in the vestibular nuclei to any of the neurotransmitters that have been identified, namely gamma amino-butyric acid, acetylcholine (Calza et al., 1989) or glutamate (Smith & Darlington, 1991). Increased neurotransmitter release into deafferented nuclei from the remaining inputs has also been postulated as a mechanism of compensation (Errington, Lynch & Bliss, 1987). Moreover, it has been demonstrated that vestibular nuclei neurones can generate resting activity *in vitro* and in isolated slices, suggesting the presence of intrinsic membrane properties which may explain the recovery of function (Darlington, Smith & Hubbard, 1989).

In the case of bilateral vestibular loss of function, giving rise to oscillopsia, the cervico-ocular reflex has been implicated in recovery of function (Dichgans, Nauck & Wolpert, 1973; Bles, De Jong & Rasmussen, 1984; Bronstein & Hood, 1987). Other workers have suggested that slip of the retinal image in this condition may be compensated for by central visual mechanisms as occurs in congenital nystagmus (Buchelle, Brandt & Degner, 1983) and ocular motor palsies (Wist, Brandt & Krafczyk, 1983). This latter hypothesis would be in keeping with the reduced optokinetic response seen in patients with longstanding vestibular failure (Zee, Yee & Robinson, 1976).

In practical terms, vestibular compensation is similar to the well-recognised phenomenon of vestibular habituation. Both physiological phenomena tend to oppose inappropriate responses induced either by contradictory information arising from the vestibular and/or other sensory organs, such as vision or proprioception, or as a result of exposure to an unusual motion environment. The aim, therefore, of vestibular rehabilitation is to expedite compensation by facilitating habituation together with balance retraining. *Habituation therapy* relies on the plasticity of the central nervous system specifically to recalibrate vestibulo-ocular and vestibulo-spinal responses, whereas balance retraining involves *sensory substitution* and utilises the redundancy within the balance system in Man to promote alternative balance strategies (Table 2.2).

**Table 2.2** Compensatory mechanisms

---

*Adaptation/habituation/plasticity:*
   Recalibration of the gain of the vestibular reflexes

*Substitution:*
   Other sensory inputs (for example, vision, cervical proprioception)
   Strategies based on prediction/anticipation
   Alternative motor responses (for example, saccades)

---

## Clinical correlates of compensation

As noted above, a number of factors have been identified as being of relevance in the failure of compensation or intermittent decompensation, including impairment of sensory inputs, neurological damage, particularly to the brainstem/cerebellum, and psychological factors.

In terms of developing a rehabilitation programme for an individual patient aimed at expediting compensation, emphasis has been placed on an initial assessment to identify factors, which may compromise the rehabilitation effort (Shumway-Cook & Horak, 1990) (Figure 2.5).

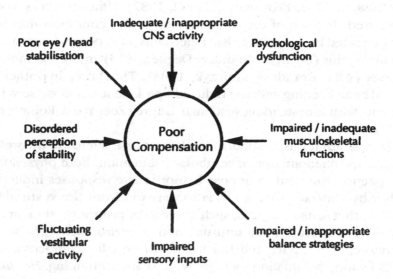

**Figure 2.5** Factors predisposing to decompensation. (After Shumway-Cook & Horak, 1990.)

Psychological dysfunction and its relationship to failure of compensation is discussed in Chapters 6 and 7. Impaired musculoskeletal function, such as arthritis, should be appropriately treated to enable active participation in the rehabilitation programme promoting vestibular compensation. In a similar manner, patients in poor physical condition should be encouraged to take part in an active exercise programme to improve their general fitness, in order to participate actively in the programme. Patients with impaired visual input should be assessed ophthalmologically to ensure optimal treatment, for example, cataract removal and appropriate optical correction of visual deficits. Inappropriate perception of stability can be improved by use of biofeedback with posturographic self-monitoring. Retraining, in terms of stance and gait strategies, is important — again, to facilitate and enhance the vestibular rehabilitation programme (Herdman et al., 1993). Inadequate/inappropriate central nervous system activity cannot be altered, but it is an important factor in determining the expectation and outcome of any rehabilitation programme based on vestibular compensation.

It is important to be aware that the central nervous system cannot compensate for fluctuating or changing vestibular activity and, thus, vestibular disorders, in which vestibular activity may acutely change, such as Ménière's disease and benign paroxysmal positional vertigo (BPPV), require appropriate treatment and resolution of acute attacks, before attempting to expedite vestibular compensation. Moreover, conditions such as chronic middle ear disease require appropriate treatment prior to the commencement of such a programme.

## Clinical presentations of failure of vestibular compensation

Figure 2.6 outlines the natural history of peripheral vestibular pathology with compensation giving rise to the asymptomatic state, but (as outlined above) this recovery process may be incomplete or, indeed, may break down, i.e. decompensation may occur after the

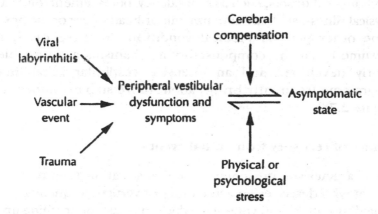

**Figure 2.6** The process of compensation and decompensation of a peripheral vestibular disorder.

asymptomatic state has been achieved. Recent work has suggested that vestibular rehabilitation is of value in all forms of disorientation regardless of diagnosis (Shepard et al., 1993; Yardley & Luxon, 1994).

In addition, there is some evidence to suggest that there may be a critical period during which, if error signals are not provided to the adaptive mechanisms and recalibration of the vestibular function does not begin, the rate of recovery and, perhaps, the ultimate degree of recovery may decrease (Lacour, 1989). The obvious implication of this finding is that when a patient suffers a vestibular deficit, active exercise stimulating the vestibulo-ocular and vestibulo-spinal reflexes should be encouraged as soon as possible. However, Shepard and coworkers (1993) did not identify duration of symptoms, nor interestingly, age, as negative prognostic factors of a vestibular rehabilitation programme. Financial compensation, head injury and severe postural control abnormalities, however, have all been determined to predict poor outcome. In the clinic, three specific decompensation syndromes are commonly observed.

### Recurrent episodes of vertigo with no interval symptoms

Characteristically, the patient presents with recurrent episodes of vertigo, which are incapacitating, frequently necessitating time off work or preventing normal everyday activities. On close questioning, the initial acute labyrinthine episode can be distinguished as being of greater severity and often more protracted than subsequent episodes, which recover more quickly and progressively tend to become less severe. The attacks can frequently be related to psychological upsets, such as redundancy, bereavement, divorce, or physical illness, such as influenza, minor head injury or the onset of some other general medical condition. In these cases, it is presumed that the compensatory mechanisms are unstable or poorly developed and an intensive vestibular rehabilitation programme frequently brings about more stable compensation (Figure 2.7).

### Failure of recovery from initial event

The characteristic presentation in this situation (Figure 2.8) is a patient who describes an acute onset of vertigo, frequently accompanied by nausea and vomiting, which may last for anything up to a week. The patient usually acknowledges that the acute vegetative symptoms abate and the vertigo has lessened, but reports that it is still profoundly disturbing and has prevented a return to normal

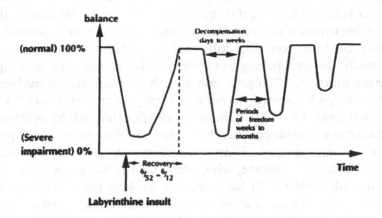

**Figure 2.7** The decompensation syndrome characterised by no interval symptoms.

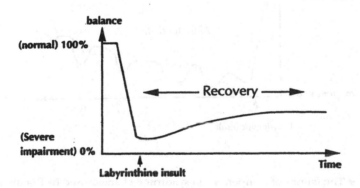

**Figure 2.8** The failure of compensation syndrome characterised by progressive, but incomplete recovery.

activity. In some patients, the recovery may be more marked with much milder symptoms, but frequently these are still described as sufficiently disconcerting to prevent normal occupational and social function. In this situation, it is important to check the various factors highlighted in Figure 2.5 to ensure that there are no compounding conditions which may be precluding recovery. An active rehabilitation programme should then be commenced (Chapter 9).

## Persistent fluctuation of symptoms after initial episode

The third common pattern of failure of recovery from a vestibular disorder is that following the acute onset of a vestibular illness, the patient improves but then relapses and subsequently continues a pattern of improvement followed by relapses (Figure 2.9). Frequently, the patient begins to become disheartened as, although there is a mild overall improvement, each step forward seems beset by three steps backwards in terms of symptomatic recovery. As in those patients who fail to recover, factors that might preclude vestibular compensation must be excluded. Moreover, it is important to ensure that there is no intermittent vestibular component, such as Ménière's disease, which has been misdiagnosed, or the presence of BPPV, which has been overlooked, for which specific treatment must be instigated. A standard vestibular rehabilitation programme, as outlined in Chapter 9, should be undertaken.

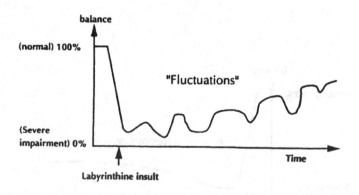

**Figure 2.9** The failure of compensation syndrome characterised by fluctuating symptoms.

In conclusion, the precise mechanisms of vestibular compensation in humans remain poorly defined. Many of the data that are available have come from studies on cats, monkeys and guinea-pigs and are incomplete, inconclusive and, at worst, contradictory (Smith & Curthoys, 1988). Inevitably, one of the difficulties in understanding vestibular compensation is the multiple number of inputs to the vestibular nuclei, which may directly or indirectly affect both the vestibulo-ocular and/or the vestibulo-spinal activity. Notwithstanding this, in practical terms, it is clear that vestibular rehabilitation programmes facilitate and expedite symptomatic recovery from vestibular lesions. There is some evidence to suggest that disorientation from other causes may also benefit from an active rehabilitation programme.

# Chapter 3
# Disorders of balance

ROSALYN A DAVIES

## Introduction

The term 'dizziness', as used both by the medic and the layman, is a non-specific term and includes vague symptoms of disorientation and lightheadedness as well as the more clear-cut symptoms of vertigo and imbalance. These may, none the less, all be symptoms of disturbance in the vestibular system and represent a final common pathway for a variety of pathological lesions. The range of causes of dizziness includes minor peripheral vestibular dysfunction as well as more centrally placed lesions, i.e. acoustic neuroma and multiple sclerosis, but also includes hyperventilation or even wearing bifocal lenses for the first time. To simplify the approach to identifying the site and, ultimately, the aetiology of the lesion, it is helpful to bear in mind a basic understanding of the sensorimotor physiology under-lying the maintenance of balance.

Pathological lesions in any of the three main stabilising sensory pathways, i.e. the vestibular, proprioceptive and visual systems, may result in dizziness. Because of the capacity of the central nervous system to compensate for peripheral lesions, an isolated lesion in one of these systems is unlikely to cause persistent dizziness. However, when two or more of these stabilising systems are affected, the capacity of the central nervous system to compensate may be restricted. Lesions affecting the brainstem integrating centres at the level of the vestibular nuclei or lesions in higher centres modulating the basic vestibulo-ocular and vestibular-spinal reflexes may also result in dizziness. Similarly, lesions affecting effector pathways, i.e. the pyramidal or extra-pyramidal pathways or lesions of the musculo-skeletal system, may also result in poor balance.

# Mechanisms of dizziness

Thus, to identify the cause of dizziness appropriately, a detailed medical history must be obtained, including questions related to the cardiovascular, musculo-skeletal and ophthalmological systems, in addition to a detailed history of otological and any neurological symptoms. It is also important to identify the characteristics of the dizziness the patient is describing.

## Vertigo

Defined as an illusion of movement, vertigo not only includes sensations of rotation either of the environment or within the head itself, but also includes sensations of being pulled downwards or sideways or of the room tilting. The sensory epithelium of the cristae of the semicircular canals and cupulae of the otolith organs detect angular and linear accelerations of the head, respectively, modulating the resting discharge rate of VIIIth nerve fibres. Imbalance of tonic vestibular signals arriving at the vestibular nuclei as a result of unilateral pathology results in an illusion of movement which is usually rotational around an earth fixed axis.

## Pre-syncopal lightheadedness

This is best described as a sensation of an impending faint, and results from cerebral ischaemia. There is frequently a sense of falling and common causes include hyperventilation, a postural drop in blood pressure or a low cardiac output.

## 'Multisensory dizziness'

A term coined by Drachman and Hart (1972) occurs with pathology involving multiple sensory systems. This is frequently the pertinent diagnosis in elderly patients, with failing vision and hearing as well as a peripheral vestibular lesion, or in patients with systemic disorders such as diabetes (see below). Typically it leads to difficulty in walking unaided.

A similar situation understood best as 'sensory conflict' occurs in patients with ocular dizziness who experience symptoms of dysequilibrium for the first time on wearing glasses, i.e. physiological mismatch of visual and vestibular inputs resulting from changes in ocular refraction.

A further category of dizziness described by Baloh and Honrubia (1990) as **psycho-physiologic dizziness**, common clinically, includes symptoms such as visual vertigo and space phobia (Marks, 1981), i.e. syndromes presenting to and recognised by psychiatrists as well as neuro-otologists. These symptoms are frequently feelings of dissociation, floating, of pressure on the top of the head and are associated with other symptoms of anxiety. Included in this group would be phobic postural vertigo as described by Brandt, Huppert and Dieterich (1994).

# General medical history

On the understanding that a good clinical history of dizziness needs to include questions relating to the type of dizziness, i.e. illusion of movement or lightheadedness, the history should also include the known triggers of the dizziness, i.e. head or body movements and, specifically, turning over in bed, sudden loud noises and also certain visual environments, such as milling crowds, supermarkets, fluorescent lighting, or empty corridors.

**Table 3.1** General medical history

| | |
|---|---|
| Endocrine disease | diabetes |
| Vascular disease | hypertension, ischaemic heart disease, peripheral vascular disease |
| Infections | syphilis, borrelia |
| Drugs | anti-convulsants, hypotensive tranquillisers |
| Haematological disorder | anaemia, hyperviscosity syndromes, dysproteinaemias |
| Cardiac disease | low cardiac output (i.e. aortic stenosis, carotid sinus hypersensitivity) |

Systemic illnesses affecting multiple systems, for example, diabetes, can cause dizziness through their effects on the blood sugar level but also through peripheral neuropathy and retinopathy affecting the stabilising sensory systems of proprioception and vision, respectively. Evidence of vascular disease, such as hypertension, arteriopathy, or a history of stroke, needs to be identified and specific questioning about cardiac disease may identify a rheumatic heart lesion, i.e. aortic stenosis, recent ischaemic heart disease or arrhythmia resulting in a low cardiac output (Table 3.1). Infectious diseases, such as syphilis, either congenital or acquired, may have serious otological manifestations. A drug history should identify those resulting in ataxia as a side-effect, i.e. anti-convulsants such as phenobarbitone or phenytoin, or alternatively those with central depressant effects, such as benzodiazepines or major tranquillisers. Haematological disease affecting the vestibular system includes polycythaemia rubra vera as well as anaemia and macroglobulin- aemia.

Pathology in the main stabilising sensory systems should be sought. This will include refractive ocular errors, evidence of joint disease or peripheral nerve disease (Table 3.2) and questioning about past and present psychological or psychiatric problems may identify a compounding panic disorder or depression.

**Table 3.2** Pathology in other stabilising sensory systems

| | |
|---|---|
| Ocular | new glasses, bifocal lenses, cataracts, glaucoma, maculopathy, strabismus |
| Somatosensory | |
| • joint disease | cervical spondylosis, arthritis (hips, knees), whiplash injury |
| • sensory neuropathy | peripheral neuropathy (e.g. vitamin B12 deficiency), dorsal column loss (e.g. tabes dorsalis) |

# Otological versus neurological

In attempting to localise pathology to the neurological or otological systems, it is of value to identify associated symptoms, i.e. patients are more likely to present to the otologist with associated symptoms of hearing loss or tinnitus or fullness in the ear, but may also present with a facial palsy or disordered sensation on one side of the face. Once patients describe co-existing symptoms of dysarthria, dysphagia, loss of consciousness, tingling sensations around the mouth or hemi-sensory symptoms, a central lesion becomes more likely (Table 3.3). Typically, otological disease presents with inter-

**Table 3.3** Dizziness: associated symptoms and anatomical location

| | |
|---|---|
| Inner ear | hearing loss, tinnitus, pressure, pain |
| Internal auditory canal | hearing loss, tinnitus, facial weakness |
| Cerebello-pontine angle | hearing loss, tinnitus, facial weakness and numbness, incoordination |
| Brainstem | diplopia, dysarthria, perioral numbness, drop attacks, extremity weakness and numbness |
| Cerebellum | imbalance, incoordination |
| Temporal lobe | absence spells, visual, olfactory or gustatory hallucinations |

mittent symptoms of a non-progressive nature, whereas neurological disease may present as continuous symptoms less likely to be associated with symptoms of disturbance in the autonomic system.

The causes of otological versus neurological dizziness are legion and can be categorised into congenital and acquired, the latter being caused by inflammatory disease, endocrine or metabolic disease, tumour, trauma, infection and vascular disease (O'Mahoney & Luxon, 1996). A list of conditions appears in Tables 3.4 and 3.5 and a few examples are cited.

**Table 3.4** Otological causes of dizziness

| | |
|---|---|
| Vascular | labyrinthine/VIIIth nerve ischaemia |
| Infective | otitis media, bacterial meningitis, Lyme disease, Ramsay Hunt syndrome |
| Trauma | labyrinthine concussion, BPPV |
| Metabolic | otosclerosis, Paget's disease |
| Toxic | aminoglycoside ototoxicity |
| Autoimmune | Cogan's syndrome, Behçet's |
| Degenerative | bilateral vestibular failure |
| Tumours | acoustic neuroma, neurofibromatosis |
| Inflammatory | neurosarcoid |

**Table 3.5** Neurological causes of dizziness

| | |
|---|---|
| Inherited | Friedreich's ataxia, familial periodic ataxia, Arnold–Chiari malformation |
| Vascular | brainstem vascular disease, migraine, arterio-venous malformations |
| Infective | neurosyphilis, tuberculosis, meningitis |
| Metabolic | hyperventilation |
| Inflammatory | demyelination |
| Toxin | alcohol, anti-convulsants |
| Tumours | pontine glioma, lymphomas |

## Benign Positional Vertigo of Paroxysmal Type (BPPV)

This condition has recently excited considerable interest in the medical press because of the introduction of particle-repositioning manoeuvres. However, to be sure of managing patients effectively in this way, a diagnosis must be established by a typical history and examination. Classically, patients describe rapid spinning vertigo lasting less than a minute provoked by assuming certain critical head positions, for example, turning on to one side in bed. Frequently, the symptoms are associated with nausea, if not vomiting, and occasionally with diarrhoea. The symptoms tend to occur in clusters with symptom-free intervals of up to several months in many cases.

The diagnosis is confirmed by a Hallpike positioning manoeuvre, in which the patient is seated near one end of an examining couch while the examiner holds the patient's head and turns the head 45° to the side (right or left) which the patient suspects is more likely to be symptomatic. The patient is then rapidly laid down with the head extended over the edge of the couch (Figure 3.1) and the eyes carefully observed for the development of positional nystagmus. Frequently, if the diagnosis of BPPV is correct patients will be alarmed and frightened of this procedure as they are aware of the unpleasant symptoms that will develop with the positional nystagmus. It is, therefore, important to explain the manoeuvre carefully and emphasise the importance of keeping the eyes open, even in the presence of severe symptoms. Instruction and reassurance are vital, as benign positional nystagmus may fatigue to such a degree that repetition of the test may fail to elicit signs and thus it is imperative to obtain the optimal diagnostic information from the first test. Once the symptoms and signs have abated the patient is restored to the sitting position, again observing the eyes carefully for the development of nystagmus. The test is then repeated, if positional nystagmus is observed, to determine the presence of fatiguability, which is a characteristic of BPPV, but not of central positional vertigo. Having completed the test with head turned in one direction, the same sequence of manoeuvres is repeated with the head turned in the opposite direction.

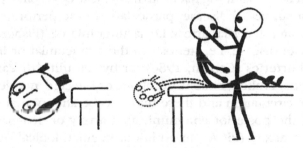

Positional nystagmus showing clinical test procedure.

**Figure 3.1** The Hallpike manoeuvre.

In BPPV, the Hallpike manoeuvre provokes rotational nystagmus directed towards the undermost ear after a short latency of between 5 and 20 seconds, but which adapts and then fatigues on repeating the manoeuvre (Table 3.6). When both the characteristic history and positional nystagmus have been seen a diagnosis is confirmed. Typical causes of BPPV include head trauma, vascular disease, viral labyrinthitis (Dix & Hallpike, 1952). The management of BPPV is outlined in Chapter 9.

**Table 3.6** Positional nystagmus

|                        | BPPV                   | Central type        |
|------------------------|------------------------|---------------------|
| Latent period          | 2–20 sec               | none                |
| Adaptation             | disappears in 50 sec   | persists            |
| Fatiguability          | disappears on repetition | persists          |
| Vertigo                | always present         | typically absent    |
| Direction of nystagmus | to undermost ear       | variable            |
| Incidence              | relatively common      | relatively uncommon |

### Brainstem vascular disease

Typically, vascular disease in the posterior circulation can lead to lesions in any part of the vestibular system, for example, the labyrinth, the VIIIth nerve, vestibular nuclei, the cerebellum or central vestibular pathways. Thus, the associated symptoms depend on the site of lesion. Vertigo in isolation is not considered adequate symptomatology to site a lesion centrally (Millikan & Siekert, 1955). Additional symptoms may include hemisensory symptoms, tingling and numbness periorally, dysarthria or dysphagia or episodes of loss of consciousness. The lesion itself may be caused by a combination of factors, including haemodynamic low flow states plus hypertensive small vessel disease, particularly in the perforating arteries arising from the basilar artery, i.e. lacunar infarcts (Fisher, 1982); by large vessel disease, i.e. stenosis in the extracranial or intracranial vertebral arteries (Caplan, 1986); or by vasculitic disease causing endarteritis. Emboli, either thrombotic or infected, may lodge in the posterior circulation and there may also be aneurysmal dilatations affecting the posterior communicating artery or posterior inferior cerebellar artery (PICA). In addition, haematological disease may lead to occlusion of end arteries, i.e. polycythaemia rubra vera and macroglobulinaemia. The pathological factors may lead to a transient decrease in cerebral blood flow with an inability to meet the metabolic requirements of the brain, i.e. a transient ischaemic episode, or to infarction and cell death (Millikan & Siekert, 1955).

### Subclavian steal syndrome

In this rather unusual presentation of vascular disease, a lesion occurs with a stenosis of the subclavian artery proximal to the origin of the vertebral artery. The arm on the side of the stenosis may be supplied by retrograde flow in the ipsilateral vertebral and during exercise enough blood can be diverted from the vertebral system to cause symptoms of brainstem ischaemia (Figure 3.2). On examination there will be a loss of pulsation in peripheral arteries in the affected arm.

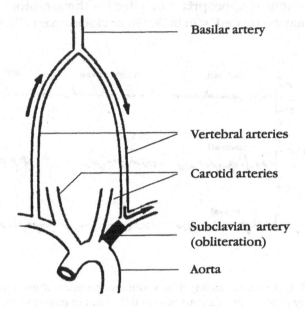

Basilar artery

Vertebral arteries

Carotid arteries

Subclavian artery (obliteration)

Aorta

**Figure 3.2** Subclavian steal syndrome. Stenosis of the subclavian artery proximal to the origin of the vertebral artery. During exercise of the left arm symptoms of brainstem ischaemia may arise through retrograde flow in the ipsilateral vertebral artery. → = direction of bloodflow.

### Downbeat nystagmus syndrome

This syndrome presents in a slightly different way to most syndromes of dizziness. Patients classically describe bobbing of vision (oscillopsia) (Bender, 1965) and associated imbalance. They may have difficulty reading signs while walking down the street, but the oscillopsia may be even more intrusive and impair reading. On examination, the downbeating nystagmus is classically seen in primary gaze, but can be increased by gaze laterally (Figure 3.3) or by extending the neck. There are thought to be two sites in the central vestibular system to cause such symptoms. Essentially, the lesion arises because of a tone imbalance of the vertical semicircular canal reflexes (Gresty, Barratt & Rudge, 1986) which may be due to lesions in the floor of the IVth ventricle or in the cerebellar flocculus. Typically, the latter occurs in association with the Arnold–Chiari syndrome when cerebellar ectopia is present, i.e. herniation of the cerebellar tonsils through the foramen magnum or with cerebellar degeneration. In addition, vascular disease and multiple sclerosis can present with downbeat nystagmus (Bronstein et al., 1987). Management depends on the aetiology, but in some cases of cerebellar ectopia, surgical decompression is indicated. When no such management is appropriate or effective the symptom of bobbing vision may be treated with baclofen or clonazepam (Chapter 5).

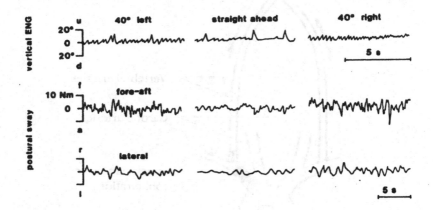

**Figure 3.3** Downbeat nystagmus: simultaneous vertical eye movements and body sway recordings in a patient with downbeat nystagmus/vertigo syndrome during unsupported stance with the head upright and fixating at a target either straight ahead or at 40° laterally. (Reproduced with kind permission of Professor Thomas Brandt, 1990.)

## Orthostatic hypotension

Pre-syncopal lightheadedness caused by pan-cerebral ischaemia has been mentioned as a mechanism of dizziness (O'Mahoney & Luxon, 1996). Orthostatic hypotension is one such cause of pre-syncopal lightheadedness. The single episode is familiar to many when, on standing up after lying in the sun, there is a feeling of faintness. Such symptomatology may be recurrent in a number of situations. Typically, the chronic use of hypotensive drugs, antidepressants or major tranquillisers may cause pre-syncope, as may prolonged bedrest and the loss of blood volume. Orthostatic hypotension is also seen with autonomic dysfunction as occurs in diabetes and multisystem atrophy, i.e. Shy–Drager syndrome (Shy & Drager, 1960).

The diagnosis is made when there is a drop in the mean blood pressure of more than 10 mm Hg on standing. It can also be provoked by the Valsalva manoeuvre. The management may require a change in medication, an increase in salt intake or in more extreme cases, fludrocortisone. As a simple measure, elastic stockings may also help to prevent pooling of blood in the extremities.

### Vasovagal attacks

In these episodes of pre-syncope the patient typically describes a sense of lightheadedness and nausea with both sound and sight receding, together with a strong sinking sensation in the stomach. Associated with the cerebral symptoms are those due to an increase in vagal tone with piloerection ('goose flesh'), sweating, a drop in heart rate and vasodilatation. Classical triggers are standing for a long time, fasting, acute visceral pain, sudden emotional stimuli or sudden severe vertigo. There tends to be a familial susceptibility among such patients. Treatment is aimed at increasing cerebral blood flow by lowering the head or elevating the lower extremities.

## Dizziness simulation battery

Drachman and Hart (1972) analysed the causes of dizziness in 112 patients (Table 3.7). Apart from showing a high incidence of hyperventilation (23%), the range of causes would not be dissimilar to a list drawn up in many neuro-otology clinics today. Peripheral vestibulopathies accounted for the majority in the 112 patients discussed (38%). This study was performed according to a protocol in which a dizziness simulation battery (Table 3.8) was used. This enabled additional diagnoses of hyperventilation, multiple sensory deficits and other neurological and cardiovascular causes to be identified. In Drachman and Hart's (1972) series, only 9% of patients were left with an uncertain diagnosis.

**Table 3.7** Causes of dizziness: major aetiologies in 112 patients* (%)

| | |
|---|---|
| Peripheral vestibular disorders | 38 |
| Hyperventilation | 23 |
| Multiple sensory deficits | 13 |
| Psychiatric disorders | 9 |
| Uncertain | 9 |
| Brainstem vascular disease | 5 |
| Other neurological | 4 |
| Central nervous system | 4 |
| Multiple sclerosis | 4 |
| Visual | 2 |
| Endocrine | 1 |
| Decreased sensory awareness | 1 |

*Adapted from Drachman and Hart (1972).

**Table 3.8** Dizziness simulation battery

* Blood pressure lying and standing (immediately + >3 min)
* Valsalva (forced expiration at 40 mm Hg for 15 sec)
* Carotid sinus stimulation for 10 sec (cardiac resuscitation facilities essential)
* Hyperventilation for 3 min
* Hallpike manoeuvre
* Cawthorne–Cooksey exercises

The aim of the 'dizziness simulation battery' was to reproduce each of the main types of dizziness. It has the specific advantage of helping patients communicate more precisely the specific conditions in which their dizziness can be precipitated. Not only will a more specific diagnosis be obtained but also patients are helped to identify the factors which are triggers to their dizziness and which, ultimately, can be managed, to decrease their sense of dizziness.

# Chapter 4
# Diagnostic tests

STEVE WATSON

## Introduction

In order to provide a successful rehabilitation service it is important to identify those patients likely to benefit from a course of vestibular rehabilitation. This chapter aims to discuss those diagnostic test techniques likely to identify this group of dizzy patients, which are applicable to a District General Hospital as well as a more specialised neuro-otology unit.

This patient group will largely comprise those whose dizziness or vertigo is caused by an uncompensated peripheral vestibular disorder (PVD), involving a lesion in the vestibular end organ or VIIIth nerve. The test techniques employed must therefore distinguish these individuals from those patients whose vertigo is of more central origin.

The purposes of the diagnostic tests are to:

- Determine whether vestibular function is normal or impaired.
- Ascertain the degree of impairment.
- Lateralise the impairment — right or left.
- Detect the site of lesion, i.e. peripheral (labyrinthine or VIIIth nerve) versus central (brainstem and more proximally).

Most of the test techniques discussed involve examination of the vestibulo-ocular reflex and nystagmus.

## The vestibulo-ocular reflex (VOR) and nystagmus

The stabilisation of gaze by the vestibular system is known as the vestibulo-ocular reflex (VOR).

Angular acceleration of the head which is in the plane of the horizontal semicircular canals causes endolymph displacement in the opposite direction to the rotation, due to its inertia (Savundra & Luxon, 1997). This results in a bilateral but opposite deviation of the paired cupulae with a change in the firing rate of both vestibular nerves. This asymmetry of neural activity is transmitted to the vestibular nuclei and results in a coordinated contraction of the ocular muscles responsible for horizontal eye movements, and hence a compensatory eye movement. The function of this VOR is to generate eye movements which are equal in amplitude but opposite in direction to the head movements causing them, in order to stabilise the image formed on the retina during head movements. When the amplitude of the eye movement is large, however, the slow vestibular-induced motion is interrupted by a fast movement in the opposite direction (saccade). The purpose of this saccadic movement is to correct errors in the direction of gaze and bring the desired object of fixation to the fovea in the shortest possible time. This combination of fast and slow eye movements is called nystagmus (see Figure 4.1). The speed of the slow phase of these compensatory eye movements relates directly to the activity of the vestibular system, and therefore the parameter usually measured is the velocity of the slow phase of the nystagmus.

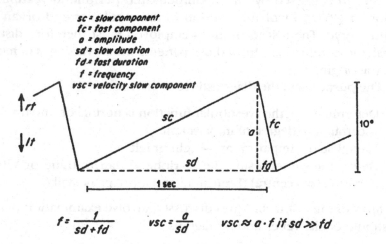

$$f = \frac{1}{sd + fd} \qquad vsc = \frac{a}{sd} \qquad vsc \approx a \cdot f \text{ if } sd \gg fd$$

**Figure 4.1** Electronystagmography (ENG) recording of nystagmus. Time is shown on the x axis, eye position on the y axis. This recording is of left-beating nystagmus, with the rapid eye movement to the left displayed as a downward pen deflection and the slower eye movement to the right being displayed as an upwards pen deflection. The velocity of the slow phase can be measured as indicated. (From: RW Baloh & V Honrubia, 1990, Clinical Neurophysiology of the Vestibular System. Reproduced with permission).

Nystagmus may also occur in the absence of any head movement. This can be physiological (for example, optokinetic nystagmus (OKN), see below) or pathological. Pathological nystagmus may be due to an imbalance in the activity arising from the right and left vestibular organs, or due to other more complex central neurological disorders. This may be spontaneous or gaze-evoked nystagmus (Davies & Savundra, 1996).

In order to quantify and document the VOR it is necessary to record eye movements.

## Recording of eye movements by use of electronystagmography (ENG)

The recording of eye movements is most commonly achieved by use of a technique known as electronystagmography (ENG) (or electro-oculography (EOG)). This is made possible because a DC electric potential exists between the retina (negative) and the cornea (positive) of the eyeball (Davies & Savundra, 1996). This potential can be picked up by placing silver chloride electrodes on the surface of the skin near the eye. As the eye moves towards the electrode the potential recorded becomes more positive, and vice versa. Given the small eye movements recorded, this change is virtually linear at approximately 40 mV/°. Horizontal eye movements are recorded by placing electrodes at the outer canthus of each eye, in line with the pupils (Figure 4.2). Other electrode configurations can record vertical eye movements (Kileny, 1985), and multiple channel recordings

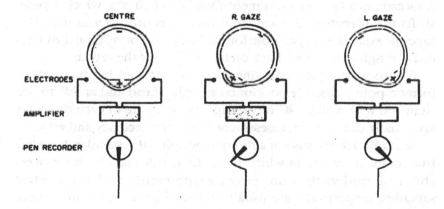

**Figure 4.2** Electronystagmography (ENG) recording of eye movements. The potential difference across the eyeball is picked up by electrodes and fed into an amplifier. Right gaze will result in a change in the potential recorded by the electrodes and an upwards pen deflection (centre) and left gaze will result in a downwards pen deflection (right). (From: RW Baloh & V Honrubia, 1990, Clinical Neurophysiology of the Vestibular System. Reproduced with permission).

can provide information concerning separate and multi-directional eye movements. For most purposes bi-temporal horizontal recording is sufficient.

The potential from the eye is fed into a pre-amplifier, amplifier and galvanometer, and a hard copy of the eye movement trace is then produced using a simple chart recorder or a more complex computerised system.

# Simple battery of ENG tests

## Calibration

Calibration is crucial to any eye movement recording and the pen deflection per degree of eye movement must be accurately known. To achieve this, fixation points are usually used, subtending a known angle in the patient's visual field. Transference of gaze from one to the other will then result in an accurately defined eye movement, and the gain of the recording apparatus can then be adjusted to provide a predetermined pen deflection (usually 1 mm/°). As the paper speed is also known (usually 10 mm/sec), eye movement velocity measurements can then be made. Conventionally, an upward pen deflection should correspond to an eye movement to the right, and a downward deflection, to the left. This process of calibration also allows a basic assessment of saccadic eye movement.

## Saccades

A saccade is a fast eye movement $(300°s^{-1} - 600°s^{-1})$, which rapidly shifts the direction of gaze from one direction to another. The saccadic system is responsible for the fast phase of vestibular nystagmus, bringing the image back on to the fovea of the retina.

Saccades are tested by asking the patient to look between sets of fixation points (usually positioned straight ahead and at 30° to the right and left) while ENG recording. Five saccades in each direction are usually sufficient for assessment of latency, accuracy and velocity.

Saccadic accuracy is not altered in peripheral vestibular disorder. Inaccurate saccades, in which the patient will initially either overshoot or undershoot the target (hypermetric and hypometric saccades, respectively) are usually followed by one or more corrective saccades. This can occur with cerebellar, brainstem and other central nervous system disorders (Kayan, 1987; Davies & Savundra, 1996).

The velocity of the saccades can also be measured. Measurements in the range of $360°s^{-1} - 440°s^{-1}$ can be considered normal for a jump of 30°. Abnormally slow saccades are often a sign of CNS disorders. A slow reaction time has also been observed in widespread neuro-degenerative disease, although it is important to first assess the level of patient concentration.

## Smooth pursuit eye movement

This is the second main type of eye movement, and is also known as a tracking eye movement. The eyes should accurately follow a smoothly moving object up to a velocity of 60–70° s⁻¹ at a frequency of 1–1.5 Hz. At higher target velocities, which cannot be matched by smooth pursuit, corrective 'catch-up' saccades are seen.

The patient is asked to track a smoothly moving target. Often, a laser target is used, and the stimulus is a sinusoid. If the amplitude is fixed at ± 20° and the frequency altered (for example, 0.2, 0.3 and 0.4 Hz) different velocities can be assessed. Although less controllable, a simple pendulum can be employed to provide a sinusoidal stimulus if an electronically generated target is not available.

Assessment of smooth pursuit is first evaluated qualitatively. A normal response matches the target trajectory accurately, although elderly patients often perform less well as smooth pursuit cannot match the target velocities. In addition, the gain of the eye movement can be measured, where:

$$\text{Gain} = \frac{\text{Eye velocity}}{\text{Target velocity}}$$

Although transient impairment of pursuit has been observed in acute PVD, decreased gain, or the presence of catch-up saccades leading to the break-up of the trace may be a sign of a central neurological disorder, such as brainstem compression, cerebellar disorders and diffuse degenerative disorders (Kayan, 1987). It is, however, important to recall that fatigue, drugs and alcohol may impair pursuit, usually symmetrically.

## Spontaneous and gaze-evoked nystagmus

Nystagmus which is present without vestibular stimulation is termed spontaneous nystagmus. It is important to assess this with the patient's gaze straight ahead, to the right and to the left, and also with and without visual fixation. This can be achieved by seating the patient in the dark and asking them to fixate on lights directly ahead, 30° to the right and 30° to the left, and to maintain their direction of gaze after the light is extinguished. Recording for 10 sec with fixation and 25 sec without should be adequate, as longer periods of gaze deviation may result in physiological nystagmus secondary to fatigue, even in normal subjects.

Spontaneous nystagmus appears as a regular saw-tooth nystagmus, when the patient's gaze is in the primary (straight ahead) direction. It occurs with PVD due to an imbalance in the neural activity within the vestibular nerves, due either to a lesion affecting the vestibular end organ or the VIIIth nerve. It is suppressed by optic fixation, and is usually enhanced by gaze towards the direction of the fast phase.

Spontaneous nystagmus can be rated in severity according to Alexander's Law. First-degree spontaneous nystagmus is observed *only* with gaze in the direction of the fast phase, second-degree occurs in primary gaze and third-degree occurs when the eyes are deviated in the opposite direction to the fast phase of the nystagmic response (Hood, 1984a). Spontaneous nystagmus will usually beat away from the affected side, unless the lesion is irritative. Following acute vestibular failure, the intensity of spontaneous nystagmus tends to decrease as central compensation occurs.

Spontaneous nystagmus can also have a central neurological origin. This is rare in the absence of other neurological or oculomotor signs, and there are several indicators distinguishing it from nystagmus of a peripheral type. Unlike spontaneous nystagmus seen with PVD, which is usually horizontal and beats away from the affected ear, it may be multi-directional and may change with the direction of gaze (gaze-evoked nystagmus). It is usually *inhibited* or unchanged by the removal of optic fixation. This basic method of differentiating peripheral from central nystagmus allows appropriate neurological referral. The reader is referred to standard texts for more detailed descriptions of congenital, ocular central neurological/vestibular forms of nystagmus, which may be identified on electronystagmography (Leigh & Zee, 1991).

# Testing of horizontal semicircular canal function

In order to provide more diagnostic information concerning the vestibular organs, it is necessary to stimulate the semicircular canals and record the resultant eye movements. The only procedure available to most clinics to achieve this is the caloric test.

## The caloric test

This is the only routine diagnostic test in which right and left semi-circular canal function can be examined separately. This is its major advantage. However, it also has the advantage of being relatively cheap, and therefore widely available. Its drawbacks include poor patient acceptability, and the fact that a high degree of competence is necessary to perform the test and analyse test results adequately.

The patient is positioned on a couch, with the head at an angle of 30° to the horizontal, to bring the horizontal semicircular canal into vertical alignment (see Figure 4.3). A thermal stimulus is applied to the endolymph, by irrigating the outer ear canal with cool and warm water. This is thought to induce convection currents and hence a flow of endolymph. This will result in cupular deflection and a corresponding modification of the neuralactivity within the vestibular nerve (Fitzgerald & Hallpike, 1942).

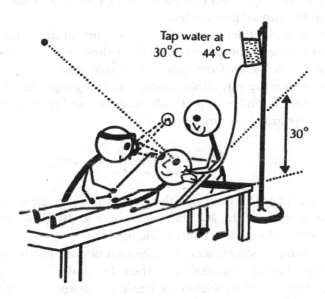

**Figure 4.3** The Fitzgerald and Hallpike caloric test position. The patient lies on a couch with the head inclined at 30°, bringing the horizontal semicircular canal into the vertical plane and allowing thermal stimulation to effect maximum displacement of the endolymph in the horizontal canal. Visual fixation is allowed and the resulting eye movements observed directly.

As only one ear is irrigated at a time, this will create an asymmetry in vestibular activity and hence stimulate the VOR. Nystagmus will result, beating towards the 'warmer' ear. The maximum intensity of this nystagmus occurs approximately 10–12 sec after cessation of the irrigation, and the response usually persists for 90–120 sec with fixation. The eye movement response is observed directly with and without fixation using Frenzel glasses or an infra-red viewer in the dark. Alternatively, the test can be performed with ENG recording.

The Fitzgerald–Hallpike test technique involves irrigating both ears in turn with water 7° below and 7° above body temperature (30°C and 44°C, respectively). The optimal order of testing is a controversial issue. However, at The National Hospital left cool–right cool–left warm–right warm is the order of choice; because the cool irrigation tends to have greater acceptability for most patients. The four irrigations will provide information concerning right and left beating nystagmus, from both ears. The strength of response can be ascertained in each case, either by measuring the duration of the nystagmic response (i.e. when direct observation is employed) or the maximum slow phase velocity (with ENG recording). Two comparisons can then be made, canal paresis and directional preponderance.

A canal paresis, which is a reduction in the semicircular canal function of one ear compared with the other, is determined by comparing the reaction from one ear to that obtained from the other. The following equation, known as the Jongkees formula (Jongkees, Maas & Philipzoon, 1962), may be used to determine a percentage asymmetry in function:

$$\text{Canal paresis (\%)} = \frac{(L_{30} + L_{44}) - (R_{30} + R_{44})}{L_{30} + L_{44} + R_{30} + R_{40}} \times 100$$

where, for example, $L_{30}$ indicates the strength of the response arising from irrigation of the left ear with water at 30°C. A negative value indicates reduced function on the left.

A directional preponderance indicates a tendency for the eyes to deviate in one direction more than in the other and is a reflection of asymmetric neural activity within the vestibular system as a whole. It is determined by comparing the right-beating nystagmus to that beating to the left. The following equation is useful:

$$\text{Directional preponderance (\%)} = \frac{(L_{30} + R_{44}) - (R_{30} + L_{44})}{L_{30} + L_{44} + R_{30} + R_{40}} \times 100$$

For both the above measures it is first necessary to establish a normal range, ideally in the individual clinic setting with the equipment to be used.

The effect of optic fixation can also be assessed as part of the caloric test. In normal subjects or those with a peripheral lesion, optic fixation will inhibit the nystagmic response (Davies & Savundra, 1996). Failure to inhibit with fixation is the sign of central neurological dysfunction. The optic fixation index can be calculated thus:

$$OFI = \frac{maxSPV_{fixation}}{maxSPV_{without\ fixation}}$$

where maxSPV is the maximum slow phase velocity of the nystagmus. An OFI of <0.8 tends to indicate a peripheral/normal type response; conversely, if the OFI is ⩾0.8 a more central cause is indicated.

The reliability of the caloric test results may be improved by checking for the flush sign after each warm irrigation. This involves performing otoscopy, a reddened tympanic membrane indicating successful irrigation. In addition, evidence suggests that the gain of the VOR may be influenced by the arousal or anxiety level of the patient, therefore test instructions must be modified to take this into account. A highly anxious patient should be calmed if possible, conversely an inattentive patient should be given an alerting task (for example, counting, mental arithmetic) in order to avoid suppression of the response. Where there is a perforation of the tympanic membrane or ear infection, water irrigation is contra-indicated. Figure 4.4 shows a patient undergoing the caloric test.

## More specialised tests

Those patients who appear to have central signs on testing, or for whom routine testing has failed to elucidate a diagnosis, may be referred to a specialised centre for further tests. The more commonly avaliable of these will be described.

### Optokinetic nystagmus (OKN)

Optokinetic nystagmus is a reflex oscillation of the eyes caused by consecutive movements in the visual field (Hood, 1984b), such as a pattern of stripes moving across the field of vision. It is tested as part of the ENG visual test battery. Usually a large curtain, with a pattern of vertical stripes, is rotated around the subject, who has

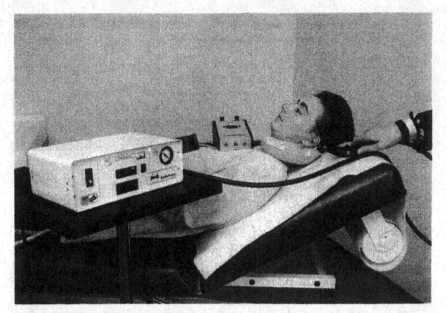

**Figure 4.4** A patient undergoing the caloric test. (From Davis & Savundra, 1997 with kind permission)

been asked to look straight ahead. A slow eye movement should result, interrupted by corrective saccade (fast phase). The curtain is rotated to the left and right in succession and the results obtained analysed for gain and symmetry. An abnormal OKN response may have unilaterally or bilaterally reduced gain (or be absent completely), may have irregularities in the rhythm or amplitude, or very rarely may reverse (in which the slow tracking eye movement is in the opposite direction to the motion of the stimulus (Yee et al, 1982)).

Although acute PVD with spontaneous vestibular nystagmus may result in an asymmetric OKN response, OKN abnormalities are usually suggestive of brainstem compression, cerebellar disorders or other CNS disorders (Yee et al., 1982).

**Rotatory chair tests**

These tests are often only available to the specialised balance clinic. Both horizontal semicircular canals are stimulated by rotating the patient in a rotating chair. ENG is used to record and analyse the resulting eye movements.

In the sinusoidal VOR test the patient is oscillated about the vertical earth fixed axis. A sinusoidal movement is used, commonly with a frequency of 0.2 Hz and a peak velocity of $30°s^{-1}$. Patients are seated in the dark, and instructed to keep their eyes open. Movement to the right induces right-beating nystagmus, and to the left,

left-beating nystagmus. The slow phase velocities of these responses are compared for symmetry. A significant imbalance usually indicates a directional preponderance (DP). The following equation can be used to calculate the DP, by use of maximum slow phase velocity measurements:

$$DP\ (\%) = \frac{CW - CCW}{CW + CCW} \times 100$$

where CW is the response in the clockwise direction, CCW that in the counter-clockwise direction.

The effect of optic fixation is also assessed. In this case the patient is asked to fixate on a light moving with the chair. The ocular response should be abolished completely at the frequency and peak velocity noted above. Failure to suppress this response is a sign of CNS (usually cerebellar) involvement (Davies & Savundra, 1997).

The other main test available with a rotating chair is the impulsive rotation (or step velocity) test. Here, the patient is accelerated rapidly from rest to a velocity of $60°s^{-1}$, in less than 1 sec. Nystagmus, beating in the direction of rotation, is induced. This will subside, however, as the chair is rotated at a constant velocity, owing to the semicircular canals being responsive to acceleration, not velocity. After the nystagmus has subsided the chair is stopped with the same rapid deceleration. Nystagmus will reappear, beating in the opposite direction. This is repeated with the chair moving in the opposite starting direction, hence four nystagmic responses are obtained. The durations or maximum slow phase velocities of each of these can be measured, and comparison of the two right-beating responses with the two left-beating responses can give information concerning the presence of a directional preponderance:

$$DP\ (\%) = \frac{(R_{start} + L_{stop}) - (L_{start} + R_{stop})}{R_{start} + L_{stop} + L_{start} + R_{stop}} \times 100$$

where, for example, $R_{start}$ is the strength of the response as the chair starts to rotate to the right.

Rotary tests are less provocative than the caloric test, and hence may have greater patient acceptability. They are particularly valuable, if caloric test results are not available, although their localising value is limited as both vestibular organs are stimulated simultaneously.

All of the tests of semicircular canal function so far mentioned stimulate the horizontal canal only. The Hallpike manoeuvre, which

should be routinely employed as part of the clinical examination of
the dizzy patient to test for benign paroxysmal positional vertigo
(BPPV), stimulates the utricular otolith organ and posterior semicircular canal. The patient is moved rapidly from sitting to a head-
hanging position, with the head 30° below the horizontal. The
patient is tested with the head turned 45° to the right and left. Any
resulting positional nystagmus is observed directly, with fixation as
removal of fixation with Frenzel glasses has been found to induce
nystagmus in a significant proportion of normal subjects. Direction
fixed, transient, fatiguable nystagmus, beating torsionally towards
the undermost ear, is common with BPPV (see Chapter 3).

## Summary

Most departments will have access to an ENG chart recorder, fixation points, some type of smooth pursuit stimulus and caloric tanks.
These allow saccades, spontaneous and gaze-evoked nystagmus,
smooth pursuit eye movement and the caloric response to be
assessed. These tests, in addition to the Hallpike manoeuvre,
should be adequate, with experience, to determine the site of
vestibular pathology in most cases and to identify those patients
with an uncompensated peripheral vestibular disorder suitable for
vestibular rehabilitation.

# Chapter 5
# Modes of treatment of vestibular symptomatology

LINDA M LUXON

The management of vertigo must be based on an accurate diagnosis. As outlined in Chapter 3, three main groups of disorders giving rise to dysequilibrium can be identified: general medical, neurological and otological, with a few other disorders, such as visual vertigo, cervical vertigo and the multisensory dizziness syndrome, falling outside this classification. A full history and examination will usually point the examiner into the correct area for further investigation, but inevitably there is some overlap (Figure 5.1), inasmuch as diffuse cerebrovascular disease may give both neurological and neuro-otological abnormalities and general medical disorders, such

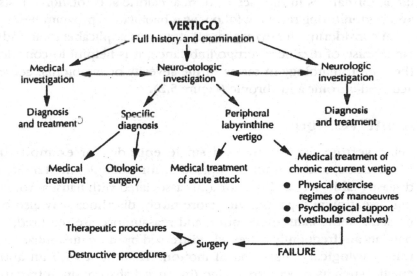

**Figure 5.1** The management of vertigo.

as diabetes mellitus and hyperviscosity syndromes, may give rise to labyrinthine and/or central vestibular dysfunction. However, specific general medical and neurological disorders should be treated appropriately and are not the remit of this chapter.

Patients with persistent dizziness/vertigo/dysequilibrium, with abnormalities on standard neuro-otological investigations fall into two main categories. The first is those with specific diagnoses (such as Ménière's disease and acoustic neurinomata) for whom standard, well-documented treatment regimes are recognised. In the case of central vestibular disorders, although the underlying aetiology may be identifiable (for example, cerebellar degeneration, multiple sclerosis), specific therapy is not always available. The second main group of cases are those of peripheral labyrinthine pathology, in whom adequate compensation does not always take place and chronic vestibular symptoms are the overriding clinical problem requiring management.

It is important to emphasise that standard vestibular tests (caloric and rotational tests) assess only horizontal semicircular canal function, at relatively low stimulus frequencies. Thus, vestibular pathology in the vertical canals, or the otolith organs or, indeed, in the horizontal semicircular canals, in the elements responsive to high-frequency stimulation, may remain undetected, despite extensive investigation. O'Leary and Davis (1994) have recently described the vestibular auto-rotation test, which allows an assessment of high-frequency stimulation of both the horizontal and vertical semicircular canals. This technique has proved of value both in identifying vestibular abnormalities in the face of normal caloric and rotational tests, and in monitoring recovery, following rehabilitation programmes.

In considering the management strategies applicable to an individual case of dizziness/vertigo/imbalance, it is helpful to consider the symptomatology in terms of the severity of symptoms: acute, acute-on-chronic and chronic (Figure 5.2).

## Acute vertigo

Acute vertigo may occur as a single episode, for example, in labyrinthitis, and as multiple episodes, for example, in Ménière's disease (Table 5.1) and is commonly associated with nausea, vomiting, sweating and pallor, and, more rarely, diarrhoea may also be present. Immediate intervention and reassurance are required, as patients are frequently extremely distressed by these unfamiliar and unphysiological sensations of motion. Treatment with an anti-emetic, such as prochlorperazine (by buccal absorption, intramuscularly or by suppository) or metroclopramide (intramuscularly) to

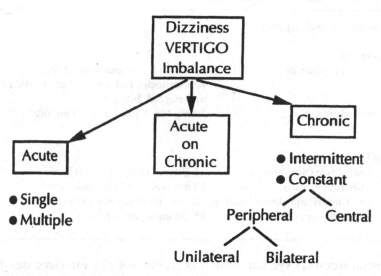

**Figure 5.2** Symptomatology of vertigo.

alleviate nausea and vomiting is essential, so that a vestibular sedative may then be administered (Table 5.2). Cinnarizine 15 mg eight-
hourly by mouth is the treatment of choice, although patients, in
particular the elderly, should be warned of the sedative side-effect
and the dose titrated accordingly. Cyclizine, dimenhydrinate and
promethazine may also be given orally or intramuscularly. It must be
emphasised that, although such drugs are of value in the management of acute vertigo, they should be avoided in the management of
chronic peripheral labyrinthine symptoms, as there is some evidence
to suggest that they may suppress vestibular activity within the

**Table 5.1** Acute episodes of vertigo

**Single:**
    labyrinthitis
      • viral
      • ischaemic
    labyrinthine trauma
    multiple sclerosis
**Multiple:**
    episodic decompensation
    migraine
    BPPV
    vertebrobasilar insufficiency
    Ménière's disease
    secondary hydrops
    progressive vestibular failure
    familial ataxia

**Table 5.2** Treatment of acute vertigo

Reassurance and support

Anti-emetics:

| | |
|---|---|
| prochlorperazine: | 12.5 mg i.m. 6-hourly or 25 mg suppositories b.d. or 5–10 mg orally t.d.s. or 3 mg b.d. bucally |
| metoclopramide: | 10 mg i.m. 8-hourly or 10 mg orally 8-hourly |

Vestibular sedatives:

| | |
|---|---|
| cinnarizine (Stugeron): | 15–30 mg orally or i.m. 8-hourly |
| cyclizine (Valoid): | 50 mg orally or i.m. 8-hourly |
| dimenhydrinate (Dramamine): | 50–100 mg orally 8-hourly |
| promethazine (Phenergan): | 25–50 mg orally 8-hourly |

central nervous system, which is crucial for the effective development of compensation and symptomatic recovery (Zee, 1988).

As outlined in Chapter 2, recurrent episodes of vertigo may occur secondary to decompensation following an acute labyrinthine insult, secondary to viral or vascular labyrinthitis, or following labyrinthine concussion, associated with head trauma. The initial insult usually recovers over a period of some weeks, but some months or weeks later the patient may suffer decompensation due to any intercurrent physical or psychological stress. During the period of decompensation, the patient may complain of symptoms of dysequilibrium, which may be acute and troublesome, or may merely be a mild inconvenience (Figure 5.3). Over a period of months or even years, the episodes of decompensation usually become less frequent and

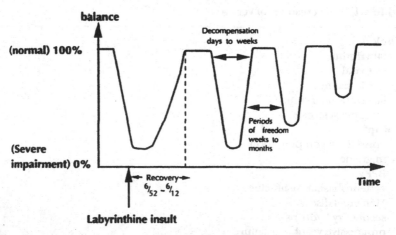

**Figure 5.3** The decompensation syndrome characterised by no interval symptoms.

less severe, such that ultimately full recovery is achieved. The process, which is dependent on vestibular compensation, may be expedited by vestibular rehabilitation exercises (Chapters 9 and 10).

## Chronic vestibular symptoms

Chronic vertigo and/or dysequilibrium may be the result of a number of different pathophysiological mechanisms (Table 5.3).

**Table 5.3** Chronic vestibular symptoms

- Uncompensated peripheral vestibular pathology
- Progressive, vestibular pathology
- Absent vestibular function
- Central vestibular disorders

The *failure of compensation* of peripheral vestibular pathology has been reviewed above (Chapter 2) and is associated with a significant morbidity, in terms of both occupational and social activities. The primary symptoms of dizziness and/or vertigo are frequently associated with secondary symptoms of psychological origin (anxiety, depression, phobic symptoms), malaise, fatigue and cervical pain, related to tension in the neck muscles. This latter symptom may result from conscious or subconscious limitation of neck movements, which are likely to precipitate an increase in vertiginous symptoms. The most common clinical presentation is of a sudden labyrinthine event of an acute nature, as outlined above, and, whereas some recovery may then take place, patients do not regain normal postural and vestibulo-ocular function, such that they persistently complain of movement-related and/or visually induced dysequilibrium (Figure 5.4). Not infrequently, there may also be an underlying complaint of constant disorientation characterised by complaints such as 'floating', 'rocking', or a sense of depersonalisation, described as feeling that they are 'living in a goldfish bowl', or that they are 'watching their life go by'. For the clinician new to this field of work, such symptoms may prompt an unnecessary psychiatric referral rather than a vestibular assessment. Patients in this category benefit most markedly from an aggressive vestibular rehabilitation programme incorporating both physical exercise regimes (see Chapters 9 and 10) and, in some instances, psychological support (see Chapters 6 and 7).

*Progressive vestibular pathology* can be particularly difficult to manage as vestibular rehabilitation is most effective when compensation for a *fixed* vestibular deficit is feasible. Compensation is not possible in the face of changes in vestibular function, as is likely to be the case during a relapse of Ménière's disease, with multiple

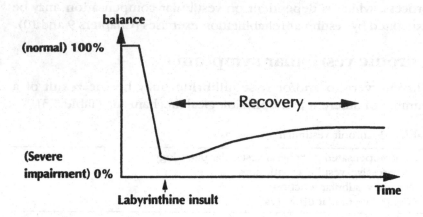

**Figure 5.4** Failure of compensation syndrome characterised by progressive, but incomplete recovery.

acute episodes of vertigo. In this situation, strenuous medical efforts must be made, by use of the standard regimes of a low salt diet, diuretic therapy and betahistine, followed by palliative surgical procedures, such as saccus decompression, if medical measures fail. In the face of severely disabling vertiginous attacks resistant to medical therapy, destructive surgical procedures should be considered. In the presence of useful auditory function, vestibular neurectomy is the treatment of choice, whereas in a dead ear, with no cochlear function, labyrinthine ablation may be considered. However, it cannot be overemphasised that before such irreversible destructive procedures are undertaken, a rigorous trial of medical therapy is indicated and sophisticated neuro-otological investigations are required, to confirm definitively the side and site of pathology. The possibility of bilateral disease must be considered.

Several points should be borne in mind before considering destructive vestibular procedures in patients with uncompensated peripheral vestibular disorders. First, psychological sequelae are common in association with vestibular pathology (see Chapters 6 and 7) and are a major factor in failure of compensation and in poor patient compliance, in following a structured vestibular rehabilitation programme. Thus, management of psychological factors and adequate psychiatric help must be provided before destructive intervention. Second, destructive procedures may be considered in a patient with prolonged vestibular symptomatology, as a result of a fixed vestibular abnormality, which is not deteriorating, but, equally, is not improving symptomatically despite attempts at vestibular rehabilitation. It cannot be overstressed that there is no reason to assume that the patient will compensate more efficiently from a total destruction of the labyrinth than from, for example, a 50% impairment. In this situation, it is more important to determine the factors which are precluding vestibular compensation and attempt to correct them.

It should also be borne in mind that vestibular compensation is less effective and slower in older subjects and in subjects with cerebrovascular disease, even in a mild form (O'Mahoney & Luxon, 1996). These factors are important in determining the outcome and in providing realistic expectations for older patients in any vestibular rehabilitation programme. Moreover, they should mitigate against enthusiasm for destructive vestibular procedures in older patients.

Chronic vestibular symptoms with constant disorientation, particularly in the dark when visual input is reduced, are characteristic of patients suffering from *bilateral vestibular hypofunction*. Patients may benefit from simple measures, such as wearing thick-soled, rubber shoes to reduce oscillopsia (associated with walking) and the use of a walking stick, to provide additional proprioceptive input through the upper limb. Takemori, Ida and Umezu (1985) have documented that patients with this condition may benefit from intensive physical exercise regimes, with the expectation of better recovery in the presence of residual vestibular function, however minor. These patients should be advised to avoid specific situations where they may be in danger, for example, swimming alone, especially underwater and standing on the edge of railway platforms and cliffs. Vestibular sedatives should be avoided to maximise the input of any residual vestibular components in these patients.

*Central vestibular disorders* give rise to chronic symptomatology, the management of which remains poorly understood and empirical in approach (Table 5.4). In patients with gait and postural abnormalities or a sense of instability or falls, such as may be commonly associated with basal ganglia disorders and cerebellar disease, physiotherapy to teach alternative gait strategies and postural control may prove invaluable in enabling them to regain a sense of confidence and improve their mobility.

**Table 5.4** Treatment of central vestibular disorders

| |
| --- |
| Retraining gait/posture/balance strategies |
| Drugs: |
|     cinnarizine |
|     clonazepam |
|     carbamazepine |
|     baclofen |

Vertical nystagmus is associated with a number of neurological disorders involving the brainstem, particularly multiple sclerosis, brainstem strokes and the Arnold–Chiari malformation. The nystagmus is characterised by persistent oscillopsia, with dysequilibrium, and often marked nausea, which is extremely distressing for the patient.

Although no specific medication has proven to be effective, there are reports of improvement in symptomatology with clonazepam and baclofen. However, the dose of the drug should be titrated by improvement in symptomatology against sedative side-effects or muscular weakness, respectively. Patients with brainstem and/or cerebellar disorders and a primary complaint of vestibular symptomatology, with the characteristic constellation of ocular motor abnormalities, including dysmetric saccades and disordered pursuit and optokinetic responses, may benefit from a trial of cinnarizine, although the success rate is low. Additionally, carbamazepine or clonazepam have been reported to be of value in individual cases.

## Acute-on-chronic vestibular symptoms

Acute-on-chronic symptomatology is characterised by acute episodes of vertigo superimposed upon background dysequilibrium. Table 5.5 highlights the commonest causes of this presentation of symptomatology.

**Table 5.5** Acute-on-chronic vestibular symptoms*

Fluctuating compensation
BPPV with underlying labyrinthine pathology
Migraine
Ménière's disease
Progressive vestibular failure
Progressive middle ear disease

*(i.e. presence of interval symptoms)

Fluctuating decompensation with interval symptoms (Figure 5.5) represents another mode of presentation of failure of vestibular compensation, in which there may be some slow progressive improvement, but the patient suffers repeated setbacks which may be associated with psychological or physical stress, such as colds or upper respiratory tract infections, or may not be attributable to any specific identifiable cause. Such patients should be managed in a similar way to any patient with decompensation, with aggressive vestibular rehabilitation, including both psychological support and physical exercise regimes.

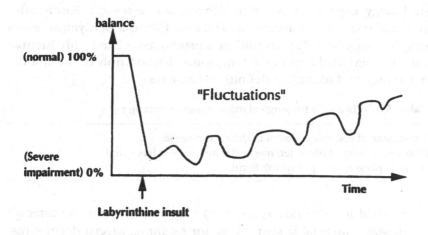

**Figure 5.5** Failure of compensation syndrome characterised by fluctuating symptoms.

BPPV is an extremely troublesome condition, despite the short-lived nature of the episodic attacks of vertigo. Although this condition is commonly idiopathic, it may also result following head injury with labyrinthine concussion and after labyrinthitis, of both vascular and viral aetiology. The management of BPPV is outlined in Chapter 9 and any underlying uncompensated vestibular pathology attributable to horizontal semicircular canal dysfunction should then be treated along the standard lines of vestibular rehabilitation.

Migraine and Ménière's disease require specific medical treatment, whereas progressive middle ear disease requires urgent surgical intervention. Idiopathic, progressive vestibular failure may present with acute short-lived, recurrent attacks of vertigo and/or oscillopsia (Bronstein et al., 1996) which should be treated symptomatically. Once the underlying condition has been treated any residual symptoms may be managed by appropriate vestibular rehabilitation. In all cases of acute-on-chronic vertigo, it is of value to correct any obvious factors which may preclude compensation and, thus, a general medical examination should be undertaken and appropriate measures put in place, such as visual correction, management of arthritis and correction of posture/gait strategies.

## Surgical management of vertigo

The surgical management of vertigo has been reviewed by Ludman (1984) and is indicated in three main areas (Table 5.6). All cases of acute vertigo should be thoroughly examined to exclude chronic middle ear disease and, if there is any suggestion of middle ear pathology, expert otological advice should be sought. Rarely, after physical trauma or barotrauma (Luxon, 1996), a perilymph fistula may be suspected. This condition is usually associated with fluctuating cochlear and vestibular symptoms. Exploration of the middle ear is required to make a definitive diagnosis.

**Table 5.6** Indications for surgical management of vertigo

Treatment of complications of middle ear disease
Improve quality of life when medical management has failed
Exclude presence of perilymph fistula

Surgical intervention (Table 5.7) may be therapeutic to attempt to alleviate intractable symptoms, for example, saccus decompression for Ménière's disease (Merchant, Rauch & Nadol, 1995), plugging of the posterior semicircular canal for benign positional vertigo (Parnes & McClure, 1991) and tumour excision for cholesteatoma and cerebellopontine angle lesions, or destructive to remove the vestibular structures and (labyrinthectomy or VIIIth nerve section) and prevent abnormal vestibular neural activity reaching the brain. Severe, recurrent, persistent vertigo, particularly due to ongoing pathology such as intractable Ménière's disease may warrant destructive surgical intervention, such as vestibular nerve section, if there is valuable remaining auditory function, but labyrinthectomy may be preferred in a dead ear, with no auditory function. None the less, such procedures should be considered only after aggressive medical management has failed, as discussed above.

**Table 5.7** Surgical interventions for vertigo

Therapeutic procedures:
    saccus decompression
    plugging posterior semicircular canal
    tumour removal
    repairing perilymph fistula
Destructive procedures:
    posterior ampullary nerve section
    vestibular nerve section
    labyrinthectomy

It should also be re-emphasised that destructive surgery should be undertaken only when the clinician is confident of good function in the better ear and is certain of the side and site of vestibular pathology giving rise to symptoms. Moreover, there should be good evidence to support the view that compensation, after the destructive procedure, is likely to be more effective than before surgery. The risk of persisting imbalance should be carefully weighed against any possible advantage, particularly in the elderly.

In conclusion, the management of a case of vertigo varies depending on underlying pathology and the presentation of symptomatology. Acute vertigo is treated primarily with drugs, whereas the mainstay of management of chronic vertigo is vestibular rehabilitation with physical exercise regimes and psychological support if indicated. The importance of a detailed explanation to the patient providing reassurance and encouraging compliance with a vestibular rehabilitation programme cannot be overemphasised. A number of situations require specific interventions, such as particle-repositioning procedures for BPPV, or specific therapy for Ménière's disease, before beginning the vestibular rehabilitation programme. Surgical intervention may be required if medical measures fail or to identify a perilymph fistula and treat erosive middle ear disease.

# Chapter 6
# Psychological aspects of vestibular rehabilitation

TINA LACZKO-SCHROEDER

## Introduction

Psychiatry and neurology are closely linked. Neurological disorders may present as psychiatric complaints and vice versa. In the chronic neurological diseases, psychiatric disorders are particularly prominent. Kirk and Saunders (1977) studied 2716 patients in a neurological outpatients' department and found that 13.2% had a primary psychiatric disorder. De Paulo and Folstein (1978) found that among neurological inpatients, 50% had emotional disorders and 30% cognitive deficits, and in more than 50% of these the symptoms continued throughout the admission.

Patients who present with neurological symptoms that have no organic basis present a particular clinical challenge to both neurologist and psychiatrist, and represent one in five of neurology outpatients in the UK (Mace & Trimble, 1991). However, they will not be discussed in detail here and the reader is referred to comprehensive texts (for example, Bass, 1990) on the subject. Neuro-otologically, the pertinent question is *'Why consider psychiatric disorder in vestibular rehabilitation?'* and this may be assessed in two ways:

- Research evidence shows that psychiatric disorder is significantly present in patients with persistent dizziness and demonstrable vestibular disorder.
- An effective treatment package addresses both organic and psychiatric components.

# Research evidence

## Prevalence studies

### Prevalence of psychiatric disorders

Persistent dizziness is a common complaint and one which is often difficult to manage. Studies in this group of patients have consistently shown psychiatric disorders to be the second most common primary cause (next to organic disease), affecting 10–25% of patients presenting with vestibular symptoms (Drachman & Hart, 1972; Nedzelski, Barber & McIlmoyl, 1986; Herr, Zun & Matthews, 1989; Kroenke et al., 1992). This is comparable with the 13% of neurological outpatients who have a primary psychiatric disorder. The higher percentages tend to occur in those who were seen in specialist dizziness clinics (Table 6.1).

**Table 6.1** Summary of research findings

Psychiatric disorder is a primary cause in 1/5 to 1/4 of patients with persistent dizziness

In older patients (>60 years) psychiatric disorder is an important contributory factor in more than 1/3

Psychiatric disorder is found in patients with vestibular symptoms, but not in those with other otologic problems, for example, hearing loss

In patients with demonstrable vestibular disease, outcome is related to psychiatric morbidity and not to the degree of vestibular abnormality

### Age as a factor

In the above studies, the patients presenting with dizziness tended to be mostly female (average 60%) and middle-aged (late 40s to early 60s). In an age- and sex-matched community study looking at patients at a geriatric dizziness clinic (>60 years), Sloane, Hartman and Mitchell (1994) found that psychiatric disorder was a primary cause in only 3%, but a contributory cause in 34.5%. This apparent age-related difference may be a reflection of the accepted importance and awareness of liaison psychiatry in geriatric medicine; the earlier pick-up rate of psychiatric disorders by the combined general clinics will select a more 'organic' population for the specialist clinic.

## Outcome study

The above studies describe a significant proportion of patients presenting with persistent dizziness who have a primary psychiatric disorder to account for their symptoms rather than vestibular disease. However, for professionals involved in vestibular rehabilitation, it is the outcome of patients who have demonstrable vestibular disease that is of greater interest, and factors affecting that outcome are important in clinical management. As demonstrated above, psychiatric factors are obviously important in the genesis of the symptoms and they may be expected to play a role in maintaining the dizziness. Following this supposition, a recent outcome study at the National Hospital (Eagger et al., 1992) reported the psychiatric morbidity in patients with demonstrable vestibular disease. Fifty-four such patients were followed up between 3 and 5 years after initial referral. They were asked to assess their dysequilibrium and psychiatric symptoms subjectively by self-rating questionnaires and a further battery of neuro-otological tests and standardised psychiatric interview schedules were performed in the hospital setting.

A third of the patients reported complete recovery at follow-up and a further third had experienced some improvement. The remainder reported no improvement, or a worsening of symptoms. Two-thirds of patients had reported psychiatric symptoms during the 3–5 years, although only 50% rated above the cut-off point for significant psychiatric disturbance when interviewed. Patients with classical labyrinthine symptoms had more severe canal paresis than the rest, but the degree of abnormality in the neuro-otological tests was unrelated to outcome or psychiatric morbidity. However, residual vestibular symptoms were related to psychiatric morbidity which, in turn, was related to measures of anxiety, perceived stress and previous psychiatric illness.

Thus, the patients who had high levels of anxiety, perceived stress and previous psychiatric illness and who reported psychiatric disorder during the follow-up period, did worse than those without these complications. The subjective outcome reported by the patients was not related to the degree of vestibular abnormality, but rather to the level of psychiatric disturbance.

## Psychiatric morbidity and other otological conditions

Other otological conditions do not show the same proportion of psychiatric disorders. Clark et al. (1994) compared patients with vestibular disorders with those with confirmed hearing loss and found that while 20–40% of patients with vestibular disorders suffered from panic disorder or panic attacks, none of the hearing loss patients had panic disorder and only 7% suffered panic attacks. This confirmed the earlier findings of Singerman (1980) in a similar group of patients. The explanation is probably that dizziness is an extremely common anxiety symptom, whereas hearing loss is not.

# The importance of recognising psychiatric disorder

Health professionals dealing with rehabilitation of any chronic physical complaint will be familiar with the psychological reactions of patients to their condition. Mild anxiety, depression and anger are common and appropriate responses to a chronic disability, and often provide a stimulus to participate actively in a rehabilitation programme. Patients develop their own unique coping strategies and resolution of the anxiety and depression can lead to varying degrees of acceptance that the health professional can support and encourage. However, for some, depending on their psychological make-up and other external factors, the chronic physical complaint (in these cases, persistent dizziness) is accompanied by severe anxiety and depression. Life becomes a struggle and suicide may even be contemplated. Other patients may develop such intense fear of provoking symptoms that they avoid certain activities and become increasingly socially isolated and even housebound. For these patients, an awareness of the interaction between the body and mind, and early recognition of a developing psychiatric disorder, with appropriate referral and psychological intervention, will at the least enhance, and may even save lives.

### How to recognise psychiatric disorder

Research consistently shows that the commonest psychiatric disorders encountered in patients both presenting with dizziness and with established vestibular disease are:

- Panic disorder.
- Generalised anxiety disorder.
- Phobic anxiety disorders.
- Depression.

A summary of the important features of each disorder is found in Tables 6.2–6.5. Some features are recognisable as part of normal human experience. The distinction between a temporary state of, for example, anxiety, and a diagnosable psychiatric disorder, is the **severity** (usually severely affecting all aspects of life) and the **length** of the symptoms (usually more than two weeks).

Panic disorder (Table 6.2) is less commonly seen in general

psychiatric practice than the other anxiety disorders. The freedom from anxiety symptoms between attacks and the unpredictable nature of the disorder probably explains why it is seen relatively frequently in patients with persistent dizziness. As the panic attacks are not related to a particular situation, patients searching for a cause of their symptoms are more likely to consider an organic diagnosis. In patients with established vestibular disorder other disorders, such as anxiety or depression, may have been recognised earlier, and the panic disorder be put down to acute exacerbations of the vestibular disease.

**Table 6.2** Panic disorder

Recurrent attacks of severe anxiety
Not restricted to particular situations and thus unpredictable
Somatic features: **dizziness**, palpitations, chest pain, feelings of unreality
Psychological features: fear of dying, going mad
Several attacks within one month
Comparative freedom from anxiety symptoms between attacks

Dizziness occurs in 63% of all patients with somatic anxiety states (Table 6.3) and is the fourth most common symptom next to palpitations, head and muscle aches and sweating (Noyes et al., 1980).

**Table 6.3** Generalised anxiety disorder

Primary symptoms of anxiety most days for at least several weeks at a time involving:
•   apprehension (worry about future, 'on edge', difficulty concentrating)
•   motor tension (restless, fidgeting, tension headaches, trembling, inability to relax)
•   autonomic over-activity (**dizziness**, sweating, tachycardia, tachypnoea, dry mouth)

Patients with vestibular disorder may develop agoraphobia or social phobia (Table 6.4) as a result of fear of provoking an attack of dizziness or of becoming incapacitated in a public or social situation. They then avoid that situation and reinforce the phobia. The effects on the patient's life and environment (work, home, social) is marked and severely affected patients may become housebound and intensely depressed (Table 6.5).

**Table 6.4** Phobic anxiety disorders

Anxiety is evoked only, or predominantly, by certain well-defined situations or
    objects (external to the individual) which are currently not dangerous
These situations are characteristically avoided or endured with dread
Anxiety is not relieved by reassurance
Often co-exist with depression
Types:
* agoraphobia (fear of crowds, public places, travelling away from home,
    travelling alone)
* social phobia (fear of scrutiny by other people in small groups and avoid-
    ance of social situations)
* simple phobia (highly specific to particular objects, for example, spiders,
    heights, examinations, small spaces)

**Table 6.5** Depression

Core features:
    depressed mood (feelings of guilt, worthlessness, intense pessimism,
    tearfulness and suicidal thoughts)
    persistent physical and mental fatigue after slight effort
    anhedonia (loss of interest and enjoyment)
Associated somatic symptoms:
    extreme tiredness but unrefreshing sleep with early morning waking
    poor appetite and weight loss
    decreased libido
    lack of normal emotional reactivity
    mood often worse in the morning improving throughout the day
    lower energy levels
    poor attention and concentration
    marked slowing down *or* agitation

Depression is usually more easily distinguishable from vestibular disease than the anxiety disorders as the spectrum of clinical
symptoms is different and dizziness is not a major feature.
However, atypical depression may be less obvious and depression
may, of course, develop secondary to a chronic physical complaint
in those vulnerable.

## Screening tools to detect a psychiatric disorder

### Direct questioning

Most patients are willing to talk about their coping strategies and
familiarity with some of the above diagnostic criteria may help the
health professional to elicit important information about the
psychological status of the patient.

*Self-rating questionnaires*

Alternatively, a number of short self-rating questionnaires may be useful in detecting conditions that are severe enough to warrant some form of psychiatric intervention. The following have been validated in numerous research diagnostic settings and are widely used as part of a formal psychological assessment. They are acceptable, easily administered and give a score result which is useful in providing a baseline of the psychological status, progress and treatment response:

- *Hospital Anxiety and Depression Scale* (HAD).
- *Beck Depression Inventory* (BDI).
- *Fear Questionnaire* (detects phobic anxiety and avoidance behaviour).
- *General Health Questionnaire* (picks up psychiatric disorder as part of a global health enquiry).

Copies and help in using the questionnaires can usually be obtained by contacting local psychiatric/psychology colleagues.

## Managing patients with suspected psychiatric disorder

*Broaching a psychiatric referral*

Despite the advances in psychiatric treatment over the past few decades, many patients, particularly those in the age group which are most likely to suffer from chronic dizziness, are wary about being referred to a psychiatrist and are afraid of the stigma involved. Some interpret the referral as an indication of disbelief in their symptoms and feel rejected; others feel blamed or guilty, as if a psychological factor is somehow less worthy than an organic one. Many patients, however, are relieved to be able to talk about their anxiety, depression and feelings of anger and not coping. Relatives and carers may have been concerned about the insidious reduction in quality of life and welcome the chance to recognise and deal with it constructively.

Goldberg, Gask and O'Dowd (1989) have described three steps in dealing with patients who find it hard to accept a psychological component:

- 'Making the patient feel understood.'
- 'Changing the agenda.'
- 'Making the link' (between physical symptoms and psychological factors).

The approach is non-confrontational, affirms the patients' experience of symptoms, but changes the focus from passively depending on some external cause being wholly responsible to actively participating in understanding and dealing with the psychological component.

## Referral agencies

A number of different professional groups may provide help for the psychologically disturbed patient within the overall framework of vestibular rehabilitation:

- *Liaison psychiatrist*: assesses and advises upon the relevant psychiatric diagnosis, likely prognosis and supervises medication if necessary.
- *Liaison psychiatry nurse*: often dually trained in general and psychiatric medicine. Many patients find it more comfortable to speak to a nurse than a psychiatrist.
- *Specialist psychiatric nurse*: with advanced training in cognitive behaviour therapy carries out structured treatment of all the mentioned conditions and may accept direct referrals.
- *Clinical psychologist*: with both hospital and community care settings, evaluates and treats psychological disorders.
- *Occupational therapist*: usually trained in mental health care, skilled in applying anxiety and stress management techniques, with practical suggestions about improving or modifying activities of daily living.
- *Physiotherapist*: may also be able to institute a behaviour therapy programme in conjunction with a physical rehabilitation programme.

## Principles of psychiatric treatment

A number of patients seen do not have a diagnosable psychiatric disorder but do have social or other problems which have come to light. Often, referral back to the GP or the appropriate social services will be appropriate.

In patients with vestibular disease and a psychiatric disorder fulfilling the diagnostic criteria outlined above, a treatment package is useful (Table 6.6).

**Table 6.6** Vestibular rehabilitation treatment package

| |
| --- |
| Continuation with vestibular rehabilitation exercises |
| Drug treatment of the psychiatric disorder |
| Cognitive behaviour therapy |

*Drug treatment*

It is important to:

- Rationalise drug therapy (to avoid dangerous drug interactions).
- Avoid worsening symptoms (see below).
- Recall that some patients think that psychotropic drugs are addictive or 'mind altering' and may need reassurance.
- Bear in mind that most antidepressant drugs do not alleviate symptoms immediately and improvement may take 7–21 days. Anti-anxiety effects are quicker.

Virtually all antidepressants have a dual anti-anxiety effect and, thus, are useful in both anxiety and depressive disorders. One particular antidepressant drug, paroxetine, has been specifically licensed for treatment of panic disorder.

The antidepressants vary in therapeutic profile; the older tricyclic drugs, such as amitryptiline, dothiepin and imipramine, are effective but may have anticholinergic side-effects (for example, dry mouth, blurred vision, constipation, and importantly postural hypotension which produces *dizziness* on standing), which may not be acceptable and limit use. They are, however, also sedative and help patients with disturbed sleep and agitated depression. Combinations of vestibular sedatives and sedative antidepressants are inadvisable and patients must be cautioned against driving when taking sedating antidepressants.

The newer antidepressants, the serotonin specific re-uptake inhibitors (SSRIs), tend to work faster, have little sedating properties and fewer anticholinergic side-effects but can produce headache, diarrhoea, dyspepsia, restlessness and tremor in some patients. Paroxetine, in particular, which may produce dystonic reactions and rigidity, particularly on rapid withdrawal, may be a problem. Orgasmic dysfunction may also occur. However, these side-effects affect a minority of patients and may be self-limiting; medical supervision during the first few weeks is essential. The side-effects usually occur with all drugs of that group.

The above antidepressants are non-addictive. There is **no place** in the long-term treatment of anxiety disorders for addictive benzodiazepines (for example, diazepam, valium, lorazepam), and use of temazepam as a night sedative can be obviated by an appropriately sedative antidepressant dose.

*Psychological treatments*

The above drugs are often helpful in establishing a calmer mental state with restored sleep and mood which can considerably enhance life, but may need to be followed by a form of psychotherapy after the mood or anxiety state is more settled. Patients with severe depression or anxiety disorders are unlikely to benefit from psychotherapy at an early stage and it may make their symptoms worse. Patients not requiring medication may proceed directly to psychotherapy.

There are numerous forms of psychotherapy ranging from analytic psychotherapy (exploring deep-rooted conflicts) through brief supportive psychotherapy (for example, bereavement, post-traumatic) and group therapy (formal analytic or informal, for example, patient support groups) to **cognitive behaviour therapy**. This is a goal-oriented, practical approach aimed at examining cognitions (thoughts), which may be negative, false or wrongly attributed and modifying learned behaviour, substituting it with more appropriate and adaptive coping strategies (Chapter 7). It is effective in panic disorder and other related anxiety disorders as well as depression and is widely used in psychiatric practice. A previous study by members of our department has shown cognitive behaviour therapy to be a useful and effective tool in treating chronic fatigue syndrome, a syndrome also with a strong somatic component as well as significant psychiatric co-morbidity (Bonner et al., 1994). The association of panic disorder, anxiety and depression with vestibular symptoms infers the fruitful use of this therapy. Anecdotal evidence suggests these techniques are effective but a follow-up study has yet to be reported.

Finally, the essence of treating patients with psychiatric disorder and vestibular disease is to provide patients and their carers with a treatment package which can be individually tailored to their needs, which is continuously reviewed and modified and where the patient is confident that both organic and psychological aspects are being addressed.

# Chapter 7
# Behavioural psychotherapy

ALAN DAVIDSON

## Introduction

Until 1970 behaviouralists' main theoretical inspirations came from experiments with animals and small groups of human volunteers. Since then, workers such as Marks (1987) and Rachman (1977) have produced a discipline which has weathered criticisms that it produced symptom substitution or was too mechanistic or superficial. Behavioural approaches are aimed at producing behavioural change directly, rather than by analysing hypothesised psychological conflict.

The characteristics of behavioural psychotherapy are that it is problem-orientated, structured, active, directive, empirically based, short-term, collaborative treatments based on psychological methods. Studies have shown that it is beneficial for 25% of all neurotic patients and 12% of the adult psychiatric population, and the indications for this form of treatment are shown in Table 7.1.

Table 7.1 Indications for behavioural therapy

Phobic disorders
Obsessive compulsive rituals
Sexual dysfunction problems
Social skills deficits
Sexual deviation
Habit disorders
Obsessive compulsive ruminations
Marital disharmony
Psychosomatic disorders
General anxiety disorders

This is not an exhaustive list and many other psychological and psychosomatic areas are being explored in current research conducted by cognitive behavioural psychotherapists. If behavioural therapy is to be effective, certain criteria should be fulfilled (Table 7.2).

**Table 7.2** Criteria for treatment

The problem can be defined in terms of observable behaviour
The problem must be current and predictable
The therapist and client can agree on clearly defined behavioural goals
No contraindications, such as psychosis, severe depression, organic disorders
    or substance abuse, are present
The patient understands the treatment offered and gives informed consent

Anxiety is a normal phenomenon as experienced by all of us at some time or another. However, when anxiety is of such long duration and intensity as to cause handicap, some intervention is required. A psychologist, Peter Laing, developed a useful model of anxiety incorporating physiological, behavioural and cognitive functioning (Table 7.3). This is known as the three-system theory of anxiety (Laing, 1971).

**Table 7.3** Behavioural model*

Physiological arousal
Cognition:
    thoughts
    images
    emotions
Behaviour:
    what is done and observed

*After Laing (1971).

Different psychotherapeutic approaches target different systems first, but behavioural therapy addresses behavioural responses (Table 7.4).

**Table 7.4** Behavioural responses

| Physiological responses | Cognitive responses |
| --- | --- |
| palpiltations | fearfulness |
| sweating | madness |
| dizziness | foolishness |
| breathlessness | illness |
| choking | sense of failure |
| visual disturbance | impending doom |
| nausea | inadequacy |
| muscular tension | inability to cope |
| tremor | |
| malaise | |
| dry mouth | |

# Anxiety reduction

The principle of exposure involves relief from anxiety by the individual's continued contact with those situations or environments that evoke discomfort (i.e. the evoking stimuli) until the anxiety subsides naturally. Most behavioural approaches to the treatment of anxiety syndromes employ the principle of exposure to the evoking stimuli. Research by Gelder et al. (1973) shows that exposure is the agent of behavioural change.

Exposure should be prolonged rather than brief. Stern and Marks (1973) found that two hours' continuous exposure was clinically more effective than four half-hour sessions. Exposure *in vivo* is more effective than imaginal exposure (Marks, 1975, 1980). Research comparing benzodiazepines with exposure revealed that exposure was more clinically effective (Sartory, 1983; Tyler & Murphy, 1987). As stated earlier, the basis of most behavioural anxiety reduction is exposure, which entails a prolonged period of contact with the feared situation or object and this is followed by a desired consequent reduction in anxiety. This is defined as adaption, habituation or extinction.

# Rationale for exposure treatment in anxiety disorders

The following may be a helpful guide to assist in explaining the rationale to patients. It should be used with other handouts, for example, on the physiology of anxiety, diaphragmatic breathing exercises and rules for coping with panic.

The problem, first, is explaining to patients that their difficulties are related to anxiety. We all feel anxiety from time to time and it is necessary to help us protect ourselves from dangerous situations. However, the patient's problem is that he/she feels anxious in situations that people would not normally find dangerous. In other words patients have **learned** to respond to particular situations in this way. Although the symptoms experienced are very uncomfortable and distressing, they are not, in fact, dangerous. It is helpful for the therapist to explain to patients how 'anxiety works'.

As anxiety increases, physical symptoms become more uncomfortable, for example, the heart starts pounding or dizzy symptoms become more severe, a sense of faintness may occur and the patient may start to feel the beginnings of panic and fear and a sense that something awful will happen — that they may faint, collapse or make fools of themselves. The therapist should continue to explain that the patient will perhaps feel that he wants to leave this situation immediately. If patients do this the anxiety will usually reduce immediately, thus giving relief from the unpleasant symptoms. They may have done this repeatedly in the past in the feared situation, and therefore have 'learned' that by avoiding the feared situation they will feel better.

However, it must be emphasised to patients that research has shown that if they remain in the situation nothing dreadful happens, that is they will not collapse, faint or otherwise make fools of themselves. The body is 'programmed' not to allow this to happen. The initial anxiety will remain high for a period of time and will then reduce, often in a very short time. It may fluctuate a little but will never go beyond a certain level and will always naturally reduce.

In order to help patients to cope it is suggested that they tackle the feared situation gradually at a level that they think can be just about managed and as anxiety reduction takes place, it is possible to gradually increase the contact with the feared situation.

## Real life exposure

Exposure to the feared situation is the treatment of choice for anxiety disorders, such as agoraphobia, social unspecific phobias and obsessive compulsive disorders. The assumption behind the exposure treatment is that anxiety has been learned as a result of escape or avoidance behaviour in certain situations or environments. It will subside provided the person can stay in the feared situation long enough to experience anxiety reduction. The patient, repeatedly and consistently, will gradually learn not to be afraid in these environments.

Some important principles should be followed in helping the therapist to organise an exposure programme:

- The *rationale* of the treatment programme should always be explained to patients and it should be ascertained that they have fully understood this. Anxiety should be explained, together with the fright, fight and flight response. Emphasis is placed on the fact that anxiety passes as one remains in the feared situation over a period of time.
- Exposure should be *graded*. It is important to start treatment neither too high nor too low down the patient's perceived scale of the feared situation. If it is too high the patient may be too frightened to persevere and give up. This can cause him to become sensitised, that is that he has left a situation feeling anxious, which

will increase the fear of that situation. Contrarily, if the situation is not sufficiently anxiety-provoking, it is therapeutically useless as he will not experience anxiety at all.

- Exposure should be *specific*, for example, go to Tesco on Tuesday and stay there for one hour, not 'try to go in some time this week'. It is important to have definite goals to reduce opportunities for excuses and avoidance. It also gets the patient into the habit of structuring his homework activities and exposure programme.
- Exposure should be *planned* jointly with the patient. The patient should be fully involved in all treatment decisions as the ultimate aim is to make him his own therapist. Research has also shown us that patients are more likely to undertake tasks which they themselves suggest (Stern & Marks, 1973).
- Exposure should be *frequent* and *prolonged*. These two issues maximise the opportunity for anxiety reduction to take place and reduce the risk of patients making themselves worse by sensitising themselves to a situation by leaving while anxiety is high. It also reduces the length of treatment considerably as improvement occurs much more rapidly with frequent lengthy sessions (Stern & Marks, 1973). Patients should preferably do as much exposure on their own as they can, as this is much more beneficial than therapist-assisted exposure. A therapist's presence can be a major reassurance for the patient and this will prevent anxiety from being aroused sufficiently for learning to take place. Research has shown that the more a patient can do on his own, the better the prognosis (Stern & Marks, 1973). It should, however, be noted that it may sometimes be necessary for therapist-assisted exposure, particularly at the start of therapy, or if a person is handicapped, and each case should be assessed on its individual merit.
- The patient must *consent* to treatment. Each treatment should be fully discussed with the patient, who should be aware what will happen during a session. There should be no surprises or attempts to do something for which the patient is unprepared, for his own good. This is unethical, will cause the patient to lose trust and confidence in the therapist and will be counterproductive.
- Any target chosen on exposure treatment should be *measurable* so that it may be assessed objectively, whether it has been achieved or if it has been partially achieved. Examples of unmeasurable targets are to feel 'normal' and to be more 'confident'. All targets to be measured should have a setting, a time and a

duration, for example, to get on a bus on Monday afternoon and travel on it for 45 minutes. Measurable targets assist with treatment monitoring and evaluation, and give excellent feedback.

- During exposure sessions it is enough that the patient is physically there. The therapist must be aware that certain cognitive and physiological avoidances may be used by patients which neutralise the exposure experience, for example, they may just be saying prayers under their breath or even just *'Oh God please let me out of here safely'* or they may be tensing up various parts of their body, for example, clenching the fists or gritting the teeth. If you suspect that either of these is happening it may be helpful to accompany the patient to demonstrate alternative ways of coping. During such a session a therapist may well ask the patient to describe what he sees in the feared situation, or advise him in ways of reducing muscular tension.
- If patients follow the structured and directive approach of a graded exposure programme, they will feel a great benefit to all aspects of their life.

## Medication/alcohol

Patients undertaking exposure treatment should not be on any more than 5–10 mg of diazepam daily or its equivalent and should not be drinking more than 4–6 units of alcohol daily. The reason for this is because 'states dependent learning' will then take place which will not generalise to medication- or alcohol-free states.

## Conclusion

It is very important for patients to gain maximum benefit from their vestibular rehabilitation programme, that the psychological/emotional components of their symptom processes are addressed appropriately.

The introduction of a cognitive–behaviour therapy programme for patients experiencing definite anxiety symptoms and active avoidance behaviour can greatly improve their functional ability and can aid them in overcoming their vestibular symptoms and the restriction placed upon their lifestyles.

Whenever practically possible, cognitive–behaviour therapy should be routinely included in patients' vestibular rehabilitation programmes.

# Chapter 8
# Hyperventilation

ROSALYN A DAVIES

Hyperventilation may cause dizziness as a result of pancerebral ischaemia and has been referred to earlier as one of the causes of balance disorder (Chapter 3). Hyperventilation has been quoted as the cause of dizziness in as many as 25% of dizzy patients (Drachman & Hart, 1972) and clearly this diagnosis merits further consideration.

## Historical perspective

A syndrome with the clinical features of hyperventilation was first described in the medical literature by Da Costa (1871), when he described a malady afflicting 300 soldiers fighting in the American Civil War. He reported that the soldiers became breathless, felt dizzy and unable to keep up with their comrades, and experienced palpitations and chest pain. He remarked that despite being breathless, 'respiration was so little hurried'. His management of this syndrome was to remove the soldiers from active duty and recommend rest. Ultimately, some soldiers were discharged from the army or placed in the Invalid Corps. Lewis (1954) gave a similar description of a war-related syndrome, when he described 'soldier's heart' or the 'effort syndrome' following the First World War, again emphasising the presenting symptoms of chest pain, palpitations and breathlessness.

Respiratory physiologists Haldane and Poulton (1908) described the symptoms of over-breathing, i.e. numbness and tingling in the extremities, and giddiness, and Goldman (1922) recognised that these symptoms occurred in individuals who were hyperventilating involuntarily. In 1938, Soley and Shock reported that all the manifestations of 'soldier's heart' could be accounted for by involuntary hyperventilation and the resulting biochemical changes in the blood, known as 'respiratory alkalosis'. They demonstrated symptom relief following inspiration of air with a high $pCO_2$, i.e. expired air.

## Biochemical aspects

Hyperventilation is distinguished from hyperpnoea when ventilatory effort is in excess of metabolic need. As over-breathing overrides normal respiratory control, the effect of abnormal rapid respiration is to 'blow-off' $CO_2$, resulting in hypocapnia. The low $pCO_2$ level in arterial blood i.e. $PaCO_2$ compromises cerebral blood flow causing pancerebral ischaemia. Kety and Schmidt (1948) demonstrated both arterial and venous vasoconstriction by use of cerebral angiography during hyperventilation. Raichle, Posner and Plum (1970) were able to quantify this effect, reporting a 2% reduction in cerebral blood flow for every 1 mm drop in $PaCO_2$. Effects on the heart were reported when patients with known ischaemic heart disease hyperventilated and induced both coronary vasospasm and decreased coronary artery perfusion. EEG changes have also been reported with hyperventilation, i.e. paroxysmal slow wave activity. The vestibular system is similarly sensitive to a reduction in $PaCO_2$ and ENG recordings in patients who are hyperventilating have shown second-degree spontaneous nystagmus (Kayan, 1987).

The low $PaCO_2$ resulting from hyperventilation leads to a change in the acid/base balance of the blood resulting in a more alkaline blood pH. The buffering system of the red blood cells and kidney cells is activated with a slowing of the enzyme carbonic dehydratase and a reduction in the level of plasma bicarbonate ($HCO_3^-$). Depending on the degree of renal compensation for the respiratory alkalosis, arterial blood gas measurements either show an incomplete normalisation of the pH and unchanged bicarbonate levels (i.e. the initial state) or a normal pH and significant reduction in the levels of bicarbonate (i.e. the compensated state) (Figure 8.1). Renal compensation results in an increase in the urinary excretion of potassium ions in exchange for hydrogen ions resulting in 'metabolic acidosis'.

Lum (1976), in two-thirds of his series of chronic hyperventilators, has demonstrated low levels of arterial $PaCO_2$. It has been suggested that there are two types of hyperventilators, those presenting with acute hyperventilation only and those with a chronic persisting hyperventilation state (Christie, 1935). This latter group are thought to have 'reset' the medullary respiratory centre, allowing the persistence of a low $PaCO_2$ at hypocapnic

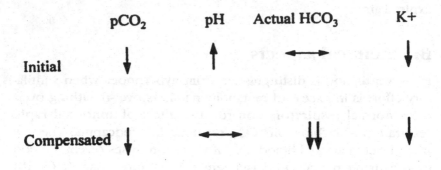

|  | pCO$_2$ | pH | Actual HCO$_3$ | K+ |
|---|---|---|---|---|
| Initial | ↓ | ↑ | ↔ | ↓ |
| Compensated | ↓ | ↔ | ⇓ | ↓ |

**Figure 8.1** Hyperventilation: arterial blood gas picture.

levels, but with maintenance of a normalised pH. This group of patients may become symptomatic with minimal exertion or mild daily stresses.

# Hyperventilation syndrome

This constellation of symptoms affecting many systems (Table 8.1) is thought by some (Magarian, 1982) to be under-recognised. Although the common features of hyperventilation include dyspnoea, chest pain and lightheadedness, some specific symptoms (for example, frequent sighing, yawning and the excess use of the chest wall and accessory muscles of respiration) are specific pointers to this diagnosis. Of the non-respiratory features, the tingling periorally and in the hands and feet are well recognised with acute hyperventilation. Syncope is less frequently recognised, as cerebral vasodilation in response to anoxia should normally override vasoconstriction due to respiratory alkalosis. Cardiovascular complaints include palpitations as well as chest pain, and gastrointestinal symptoms include a lump in the throat and aerophagia. Typically, hypocapnia in muscle tissue leads to cramp and may present as carpo-pedal spasm. The psychiatric manifestations of hyperventilation include anxiety, panic attacks, unreal feelings and depersonalisation.

**Table 8.1** Presenting signs and symptoms of hyperventilation

General:
  weakness, exhaustion, sleep disturbances, excess sweating
Neurological:
  dizziness, faintness, syncope, tingling peri-orally and in hands and feet,
  tunnel vision
Respiratory:
  shortness of breath, inability to take deep breath, excessive sighing, tight
  chest
Cardiovascular:
  chest pain, palpitation, tachycardia
Gastrointestinal:
  lump in throat, air swallowing
Muscle:
  cramps, carpo-pedal spasm
Psychiatric:
  anxiety, panic attacks, unreal feelings, depersonalisation

# Pathogenesis

The causes of hyperventilation include organic, physiological, emotional and 'habit' aetiologies. The organic and physiological causes are relatively straightforward to identify, but the recurrent hyperventilation syndromes tend to be related to reactions to stress and faulty breathing patterns (Table 8.2). In those who develop the hyperventilation syndrome, stress is the provocative factor and thoracic breathing the permissive factor. The cycle is initiated by stress, but the fear and apprehension generated by the clinical symptoms of hyperventilation maintain the syndrome in a chronic recurrent state. Christie (1935) describes two characteristic types of abnormal breathing, which match the acute and chronic hyperventilators described above, i.e. those who have difficulty in obtaining a satisfactory breath, tending to have deep sighing respirations,

**Table 8.2** Pathogenesis of hyperventilation

Organic:
  drug effects, CNS lesions, alcohol withdrawal
Physiological:
  acclimatisation, heat, exercise
Emotional:
  reaction to stress
Habit:
  faulty breathing pattern

whereas those who exhibit a full house of clinical features have irregular, but rapid and shallow breathing patterns (Table 8.3). Hyperventilation is discussed here as the primary cause of the syndrome, but many authors have drawn parallels between the presenting features of anxiety neurosis and hyperventilation (Pitts, 1969; Marks & Lader, 1973; Noyes et al, 1980).

**Table 8.3** Types of breathing pattern

|  | *Breathing pattern* | *Symptoms* |
|---|---|---|
| Normal breathing | 8–10 breaths/min controlled by diaphragm | – |
| Chronic hyperventilation | irregular, rapid, shallow breathing (i.e. thoracic breathing) | full complement of clinical features of HV syndrome |
| Acute HV syndrome | deep sighing respirations | difficulty obtaining a satisfactory breath |

# Hyperventilation provocation test

To make a diagnosis of hyperventilation, a provocation test is recommended. This is best carried out by instructing patients to describe how they feel during the test, before explaining the precise purpose of the test. Patients are asked to take 30–40 deep breaths a minute following the breathing pattern of the examiner. This should be continued for 4–5 minutes or until dizziness supervenes, and the examiner will wait for the patient to acknowledge the similarities of the symptoms induced by this breathing pattern with those experienced by the patient in other situations. By then, using a brown paper bag and asking patients to rebreathe their own expired air, these symptoms should come under control, if they are due to hyperventilation, allowing the patient to recognise the cause of their symptoms and also the possibility of gaining immediate relief.

It is essential to point out that caution should be exercised in performing this test in patients with known ischaemic heart disease, sickle cell disease, vertebrobasilar ischaemia or baseline hypoxaemia. Also, it is better if this provocation test is done in the presence of a family member or close friend, and that an explanation is given also to the accompanying person as to faulty breathing habits and the importance of converting thoracic to abdominal breathing to obtain relief.

# Breathing exercises

Normal breathing at rest is at the rate of 8–10 breaths a minute. This breathing pattern is normally controlled by the diaphragm and, when asleep, the stomach moves at the rate of 10 times a minute and, when relaxed, the rate of breathing is controlled by these stomach movements. To teach breathing exercises a half-hour time slot should be arranged and patients should be asked to wear loose clothing. Patients should sit down on a comfortable chair, placing one hand on the stomach and one hand on the chest. They are asked to breathe so that the hand on the stomach moves in and out, and initially to breathe once every six seconds with normal-sized breaths. After establishing this rate of breathing, patients should then breathe every 10 seconds pausing for longer before breathing again. When success is achieved with these breathing exercises performed sitting down, patients should then progress to the exercises standing up, and walking, at a later date (see Table 8.4).

Table 8.4 Breathing exercises

Find a spare half-hour
Wear loose, comfortable clothing
Sit down on a comfortable chair
Put one hand on the stomach, one hand on the chest
Breathe so hand on stomach moves in and out
Breathe once every six seconds, normal size breaths
Breathe every 10 seconds, pausing for longer before breathing again
Progress to exercises standing up, walking at a later date

The atmosphere in which these breathing exercises are taught is critical and it is important that the examiner has no preconceptions and is sympathetic to the condition. Where a hyperventilation state has been chronically maintained, it may take longer to change a faulty breathing pattern and patients may need to be seen regularly.

## Conclusion

Undoubtedly, hyperventilation can cause lightheadedness, but how often it is the primary aetiological factor is less certain. Many patients of an anxious disposition who develop vertigo from a primary vestibular lesion, may start to hyperventilate with the onset of dizziness, exacerbating their symptoms. This is not uncommon in patients undergoing caloric investigation, who develop symptoms of panic disorder in response to the induced dizziness.

There are many reasons why hyperventilation may be under-reported, including omission of this subject from the medical curriculum and textbooks. It may be too easy to diagnose the symptoms as anxiety, depression or hysteria with no recognition of underlying or associated hyperventilation. Another reason for a low diagnostic rate may include the lack of understanding that significant respiratory alkalosis may occur and be maintained without obvious visible breathing abnormalities. Undoubtedly, the primary complaint may mimic other disease states and the patient may present in the cardiology clinic, or the psychiatric outpatients, as well as the dizziness clinic.

# Chapter 9
# Theoretical basis of physical exercise regimes and manoeuvres

LINDA M LUXON

The basis of physical exercise regimes in the management of the dizzy patient lies in the assumption that active movements stimulating the sensory inputs required for balance, expedite symptomatic recovery from vestibular disorders. Initial work emphasised the need to differentiate peripheral vestibular pathology from other causes of vertigo before considering the application of physiotherapy techniques (Dix, 1984; Norré, 1987). However, recent work has emphasised the value of vestibular rehabilitation exercises in both peripheral and central vestibular disorders, in addition to psychological disorders giving rise to dizziness (Shepard et al., 1993; Yardley & Luxon, 1994). Until recently, there has been relatively little enthusiasm for the treatment of dizzy patients, in part because of the singular lack of success of drug treatment and the relatively small number of indications for surgical intervention. The use of exercise regimes to capitalise on the plasticity of the central nervous system and expedite vestibular compensation, both by habituation and sensory substitution, had not been fully appreciated until the last decade.

There are three main categories of exercise regimes or manoeuvres (Table 9.1). A *systematic exercise programme*, in which the patient works through a preset list of exercises, a *'customised' exercise programme*, which is tailor-made for each patient, and *specific therapeutic manoeuvres* for benign positional vertigo, such as the Brandt–Daroff exercise regime (Brandt & Daroff, 1980) and specific single manoeuvres, such as the Semont (Semont, Freyss & Vitte, 1988) and the Epley (1992) manoeuvre. This chapter will consider the rationale and use of each of these procedures in the context of an overall rehabilitation programme (Table 9.2).

**Table 9.1** Physical exercise regimes and manoeuvres

Systematic exercise programme
'Customised' exercise programme
Specific therapies:
    Brandt–Daroff exercises
    Semont manoeuvre
    Epley manoeuvre

# Rehabilitation programme

Although crucial to the success of any vestibular rehabilitation programme, physical exercise regimes must be considered in terms of an overall rehabilitation programme for the dizzy patient (Table 9.2). First, investigation and diagnosis are important in order that an appropriate rehabilitation plan may be constructed, which may then be explained in detail to the patient to ensure understanding and active compliance with the programme.

The rehabilitation plan must include correction of remediable problems, a general fitness programme within the constraints of each patient, psychological assessment (where appropriate), the consideration of any concurrent medical therapy and a long-term framework of realistic family, social and occupational goals. Within this overall rehabilitation plan the physical exercise regime used will not only reduce vestibular symptomatology but enable the patient to feel more in control of his symptoms, as opposed to feeling entirely governed by them.

**Table 9.2** Rehabilitation programme

1. Investigation and diagnosis
2. Explanation
3. Rehabilitation plan:
    correction of remediable problems
    general fitness programme
    physical exercise regimes
    psychological assessment
    medication
    realistic family/social/occupational goals
4. Monitoring/feedback/follow-up
5. Discharge

# Historical aspects

Physiotherapy for patients with peripheral vestibular disorders was first introduced by Cawthorne and Cooksey in the mid-1940s (Cawthorne, 1945; Cooksey, 1945). They recognised the tendency for patients with vestibular disorders, secondary to head injury, to drift into chronic invalidism and designed a series of graduated exercises aimed at encouraging head and eye movement. These exercises provoked dizziness in a systematic manner, on the basis of the empirical observation that patients recovered more rapidly if they were active. The original Cawthorne Cooksey exercises (Table 9.3) were performed in various positions and at various speeds, depending on the severity of the patient's symptoms, but were based on a prescribed list of exercises composed of eye movements, tasks of head–eye coordination, body movements and balancing tasks. The exercises were performed with the eyes both open and closed, in order to promote compensation using vestibular and proprioceptive mechanisms. The importance of psychological well-being was recognised and it was recommended that patients undertook the exercises in daily group lessons, in order to encourage the more reticent patients and also to identify malingerers. Moreover, patients were encouraged to encounter busy and noisy environments, as it was noted that most patients with vestibular disorders tended to avoid such situations (Table 9.4).

**Table 9.3** Cawthorne Cooksey exercises

---

**A. Resting**

Only one exercise at a time should be carried out and this exercise should be continued until any unpleasant symptom ceases. Only then, should the next exercise be started.

1. Eye movements–at first slow, then quick
    a. up and down.
    b. from side to side.
    c. focussing on finger moving from 3 feet to 1 foot away from face.
2. Head movements–at first slow, then quick. Later with eyes closed.
    a. bending forwards and backwards.
    b. turning from side to side.

**B. Sitting**

1. & 2. as above.
3. Shoulder shrugging and circling.
4. Bending forwards and picking up objects from the ground.

**C. Standing**

1. As A1 and 2 and B3.
2. Changing from sitting to standing position with eyes open and shut.
3. Throwing a small ball from hand to hand (above eye level).
4. Throwing ball from hand to hand under knees.
5. Change from sitting to standing and turning round in between.

**D. Moving about**

1. Circle round centre person who will throw a large ball and to whom it will be returned.
2. Walk across room with eyes open and then closed.
3. Walk up and down slope with eyes open and then closed.
4. Walk up and down steps with eyes open and then closed.
5. Any game involving stooping or stretching and aiming such as skittles, bowls or basket-ball.

---

**Table 9.4** Therapeutic aspects of Cawthorne Cooksey exercises

* Different body positions and tasks
* Variety of speeds
* Eyes open and closed
* Group sessions
* Psychological aspects

With the passage of time, it has become evident that the exercise regime should not be considered 'an endurance test' and that a systematic, gentle, consistent approach is more efficacious than infrequent bursts of aggressive exercises, which precipitate symptomatic vertigo associated with nausea and vomiting and deter the patient from wishing to repeat the experience. The patient should be reassured that there is no time limit on the programme. In particular, it is not a race to be completed in the shortest possible time, but, more importantly, the patient should progress at his own rate (Table 9.5).

**Table 9.5** Guidelines for patients

* Not an endurance test
* Not a race/no time limit
* Gentle, systematic, consistent approach

Despite the introduction of these exercises in the early 1940s, their use was not widespread and, indeed, there were relatively few reports in the literature for the next 30 years. However, in the mid-1970s onwards the reports of animal studies lent weight to the use of physical exercises in vestibular rehabilitation, in that visual input and motor activity were shown to facilitate the rate and final level of recovery in animals with lesions in the vestibular system (see Chapter 2). Lacour, Roll and Appiax (1976) showed improved recovery in baboons subjected to a unilateral vestibular neurectomy, if they were unrestrained, as compared with a restrained group and this was soon followed by work showing similar results in squirrel monkeys (Igarashi et al., 1981) and in cats following unilateral labyrinthectomy (Mathog & Peppard, 1982). Courjon and coworkers (1977) showed the role of vision on compensation in cats and built on the earlier work of Ito (1975) showing the importance of the cerebellum in modulating vestibular activity in response to visual stimuli. These experiments suggested that repetition of movements and positions that provoked dizziness and vertigo promoted vestibular compensation and, thus, through the physiological phenomenon of habituation, formed the scientific basis underpinning the empirical observations of Cawthorne and Cooksey.

In the late 1970s and 1980s there were a number of reports which assessed the symptomatic response of the Cawthorne Cooksey exercises (Hecker, Haug & Herndon, 1974; Dix, 1979, 1984; Norré & De Weerdt, 1980a, 1980b) and showed that approximately 80% of patients with clearly defined peripheral vestibular disorders responded favourably to the regime. All these papers were based on the assumption that vestibular habituation was brought about by the exercise regime, rendering the patient asymptomatic.

Norré (1987) took the next step forward by devising an *objective* measure of the patient's functional condition based on 19 specific vertigo-producing manoeuvres. The patients were asked to score the intensity, type and duration of vertigo produced by each test manoeuvre, rapidly performed and held for 10 seconds prior to returning to the resting position. The test manoeuvres served not only as a means to objectively evaluating the patient's symptoms but also formed the basis of the treatment regime. Patients were encouraged to perform the specific manoeuvres that produced the most troublesome symptoms (Norré, 1984). In keeping with the views expressed by Dix (1976), Norré and De Weerdt (1981) emphasised that a clear explanation of the patient's symptomatology is of value, particularly as patients tend to avoid assuming positions which are likely to precipitate their symptoms, despite the fact that it is these very positions which must be adopted if habituation is to occur. Moreover, they recognised the psychological correlates of this condition and advised relaxation therapy. Two notable differences between the Norré programme and the Cawthorne Cooksey exercises are the absence of any movements with eye closure and the absence of activities involving movement.

There has been an explosion in developments related to vestibular rehabilitation since the mid-1980s and these have hinged on four major considerations (Table 9.6):

1.  The introduction of a rehabilitation programme characterised by a holistic approach to the patient with detailed assessment of the overall physical condition of the patient in addition to the specific vestibular derangement.
2.  The introduction of 'customised' exercises aimed at developing vestibular habituation as outlined above.
3.  The recognition of the importance of the need to address the dynamic aspects of gait and balance.
4.  The development of outcome measures to evaluate scientifically the effects of the rehabilitation effort.

**Table 9.6** Recent developments in vestibular rehabilitation

- Vestibular rehabilitation programmes
- 'Customised' exercises
- Gait and balance retraining
- Outcome measures

## Current state of the art

### Rehabilitation programmes

It is now generally accepted that all patients should undergo a complete physical examination with particular reference to the musculo-skeletal and neuro-muscular systems. As noted in Chapters 6 and 7, the psychological state of the patient should be assessed and appropriate therapy commenced. The social and occupational environment should be appraised in order to modify the exercise regime to that appropriate to the patient's needs and to outline realistic expectations and goals (Shumway-Cook & Horak, 1990; Shepard et al., 1993; Herdman, 1994).

### Customised exercises

Most departments base the standard physical exercise assessment protocol on the original exercises advocated by Cawthorne (1945) and Cooksey (1945), but, in addition, specific functional deficits, related to motion-provoked or visually provoked symptoms, should be evaluated, with abnormalities of gait and postural control. These observations, supplemented by measurement made by use of dynamic posturography, allow the development of individual 'customised' exercise programmes, which may be taught most effectively by a physiotherapist, but thereafter may be practised at home with the frequency of visits to the physiotherapy department for review dependent upon the patient's confidence, motivation, progress and circumstances.

The patient should be reassured that recovery based on vestibular habituation takes time, but exercise sessions of 3–5 minutes, two to three times a day, are effective. The most effective exercises in terms of inducing recovery are those which induce an error in the vestibulo-ocular or vestibulo-spinal system and it must be stressed that the patient should work at the limit of their ability, performing exercises which cause symptoms. For example, with respect to eye–head exercises, if fixating on a target and moving their head, the patient should increase the head movements until the target is just out of focus. Exercises involving the vestibulo-spinal system can be increased in difficulty by reducing the size of the support base and by performing exercises during dynamic activities, in addition to static activities. There is evidence to suggest that voluntary motor control will improve recovery and, thus, patients should be encouraged to concentrate on the task in hand and not be distracted by other activities, such as conversation (Table 9.7). (For detailed lists of exercises for postural and gaze stability the reader is referred to Herdman (1994).)

**Table 9.7** Rationale of customised exercises

Identify tasks giving vestibulo-ocular/spinal errors
Concentration on specific tasks
Work at limit of patient's ability
Part of overall rehabilitation

## Gait and balance retraining

An important element in the exercise regimes advocated by the North American groups (Shumway-Cook & Horak, 1990; Shepard et al., 1993; Herdman, 1994) include balance and gait training during dynamic rather than static tasks. The rationale for the inclusion of such exercises is that most patients with vestibular dysfunction do not complain of symptoms when stationary, for example, attempting to stand on one leg, but complain of visually induced, or motion-induced symptoms when they are trying to live normally, for example, out shopping, cleaning their house or attempting to travel around. Thus, the aim of balance and gait training is 'problem orientated' in attempting to rehabilitate patients for specific difficulties they have encountered.

During evaluation the patient's functional balance deficits may be identified and specific retraining exercises devised to facilitate recovery from the specific problem, for example, if scanning supermarket shelves is difficult for a woman, then in the first instance she is encouraged to walk up and down a corridor moving her head up and down and then from side to side. The difficulty of this task may then be increased by placing objects in the path of the patient as she walks. In addition, patients should be encouraged to undertake the specific tasks that they find difficult as part of the retraining therapy.

The specific exercises vary enormously depending upon the individual patient's difficulties, but may include tasks such as walking backwards, side-stepping, walking in the dark on a thickly carpeted floor to reduce visual and proprioceptive inputs, and stepping forward crossing one leg over the other and backwards undertaking the same task. Some suggested exercises are shown in Table 9.8.

**Table 9.8** Balance and gait exercises

1.  Do the following exercises while standing. Stand near a kitchen counter, but only hold on if needed:
    Walk sideways 5 m. Repeat to both left and right directions ........ times, twice a day.
    Walk backwards 5 m. Repeat ........ times, twice a day.

2.  Do the following exercises while standing. Stand with a wall behind you. Have a family member stand nearby if needed. Stand on a pillow or couch cushion, for ....... sec.

    Do this with your eyes open. Repeat ....... times, twice a day.
    Do this with your eyes closed. Repeat ........ times, twice a day.

3.  Walk down a corridor and practise moving your head left and right. Keep your head turned in each direction for about three steps. Walk ....... m. Repeat ........ times, twice a day. Also repeat by moving your head up and down.

4.  Set up an obstacle course. Use chairs, pillows and furniture as obstacles. Place smaller objects on the floor that you must step over. Change the course each time so that you do not get used to the same routine. You can incorporate stair climbing, sit to stand, or picking up and carrying objects during the 'obstacle' course. Set a timer or clock yourself to see how fast you can finish. To add difficulty, have a family member shout out commands (for example, *'Turn left now'*) or throw a ball towards you unexpectedly.

5.  Walk around a darkened room in your house (carpet preferred) for ....... min.

6.  Go grocery shopping, as tolerated.

7.  Do your walking programme at a shopping centre one to two times a week.

From Herdman (1994), reproduced with permission.

## Outcome measures

In the past 10 years, since the development of Norré's 19 manoeuvres both to assess and treat vertiginous patients, there has been emphasis on the development of objective outcome measures (Table 9.9). Initially, subjective improvement was assessed (Dix, 1984), but Norré (1987) introduced score cards as noted above. Subsequently, questionnaires attempting to quantify disability and handicap have been devised (Chapter 12) and, more recently, objective posturographic measurements (Shepard et al., 1993) and the new technique of vestibulo-autorotation (O'Leary & Davis, 1994) have been used to monitor the efficacy of the rehabilitation effort (see Chapter 12).

**Table 9.9** Outcome measures

- Subjective improvement
- Score cards for specific manoeuvres
- Questionnaires
- Objective measurements (for example, posturography, vestibular autorotation)

Initially, physical exercise regimes were advocated for patients with unilateral or bilateral peripheral vestibular pathology, in whom a fixed deficit had been defined (Dix, 1984; Norré, 1987). Subsequently, vestibular habituation therapy was also advocated for the treatment of benign positional vertigo of paroxysmal type (BPPV) (Norré & Beckers, 1987, 1988), whereas Brandt and Daroff (1980) described a more specific exercise regime reportedly to disperse heavy debris within the labyrinth in this condition. However, recent work has suggested that patients with central vestibular pathology may also benefit from a vestibular rehabilitation programme (Shepard et al., 1993; Herdman, 1994) as may patients with psychological manifestations, including dysequilibrium (Yardley & Luxon, 1994).

Vestibular compensation in the elderly is recognised to be poorer than in younger people and, thus, it has often been suggested that age is a negative prognostic factor in recovery from vestibular pathology (Norré, Forrez & Beckers, 1987; Zee, 1988), although Shepard et al. (1993) have reported that age has no effect on outcome. However, financial compensation, head injury and severe postural control abnormalities have all been documented as negative prognostic factors (Shepard et al., 1993; Herdman, 1994) (Table 9.10).

**Table 9.10** Negative prognostic factors in vestibular rehabilitation

- Age
- Financial compensation
- Head injury
- Severe postural control abnormalities

The possibility of a 'critical period' immediately after a vestibular insult, during which compensation, secondary to central nervous system plasticity and adaptation to a lesion, is greatest has been raised. This concept has been based on animal experiments showing that visual input and mobilisation in the early stages following labyrinthectomy or vestibular nerve section facilitate the rate and ultimate degree of plasticity (see Chapter 2, Vestibular compensation). However, this concept was based on recovery of the vestibulo-spinal function, whereas there is evidence to suggest that immobilisation may retard vestibulo-ocular compensation less than vestibulo-spinal compensation (Jensen, 1979; Shaefer & Meyer, 1981). None the less, dynamic compensation can only occur if the central nervous system is provided with abnormal vestibular information and, thus, in patients with acute vestibular disorders it is appropriate to advise early activity.

## Specific exercise therapies and manoeuvres

Benign positional paroxysmal vertigo (BPPV) (Dix & Hallpike, 1952) is a common vestibular disorder, characterised by acute episodes of severe vertigo, on assuming a critical head position, which usually involves neck extension and turning of the head to right or left. The symptoms and rotational nystagmus may develop after a latent period of some 2–20 seconds, following which the patient becomes acutely symptomatic with unpleasant vertigo, frequently accompanied by nausea, pallor and sweating. If the critical position is held, the nystagmus adapts, but if the head is moved from the critical position the symptoms and positional nystagmus abate immediately. The condition is diagnosed by performing the Hallpike manoeuvre (see Chapter 3, Disorders of balance).

Cupulolithiasis (Schuknecht, 1969; Schuknecht & Ruby, 1973) was proposed initially as the pathophysiological mechanism giving rise to this condition. Debris from the otolith organ was hypothesised to become attached to the cupula of the posterior semicircular canal, such that on assuming a critical head position, the 'heavy' cupula became hypersensitive to the effects of gravity and a burst of neuronal activity would ensue (Figure 9.1 (A) and (B)). However, more recent work has led to the theory of canalithiasis (Figure 9.1 (A) and (C)), which better explains all the characteristic features of BPPV (Baloh, 1996).

This theory proposes that calcium carbonate crystal debris forms in the most dependent portion of the posterior semicircular canal and upon assuming a critical head position, the clot moves in an ampullofugal direction and, thus, has a 'plunger' effect within the narrow posterior semicircular canal. This causes movement of the cupula in an ampullofugal direction, resulting in a brief paroxysm of vertigo and nystagmus. In 1980, Brandt and Daroff reported complete relief of symptoms in 66 of 67 patients with BPPV, as a result of precipitating head positions 'on a repeated and serial basis' (Figure 9.2). The mechanism for this improvement was the proposed loosening and dispersion of otolithic debris from the cupula of the posterior semicircular canal, as a result of the rapid and aggressive vertigo-provocative movements. However, on the basis of the canalithiasis model, it may be proposed that these

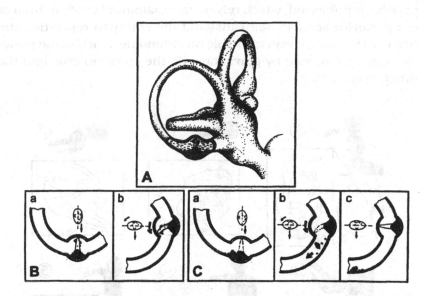

**Figure 9.1** Resting anatomical position of the posterior semicircular canal (A). The proposed pathophysiological mechanisms of cupulolithiasis (B) and canalithiasis (C) (From Brandt & Steddin, 1993. Reproduced with permission.)

repeated manoeuvres cleared the debris from the most dependent part of the posterior semicircular canal into the utricle, where the debris no longer interferes with semicircular canal dynamics and, thus, the patient is rendered asymptomatic.

The pathophysiological mechanism of canalithiasis has resulted in new developments in terms of management techniques. Single

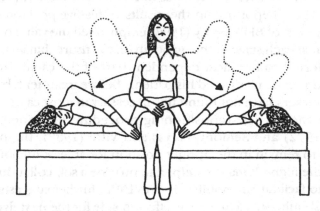

**Figure 9.2** The Brandt–Daroff exercises (From Brandt & Daroff 1980. Reproduced with permission.)

positional manoeuvres (Semont, Freyss & Vitte, 1988; Epley, 1992) have been published, which rely on the anatomical configuration of the posterior semicircular canal and the ability to reposition the head in a variety of ways to enable the offending debris in the posterior canal to migrate by gravitation via the common crus into the utricle (Figure 9.3).

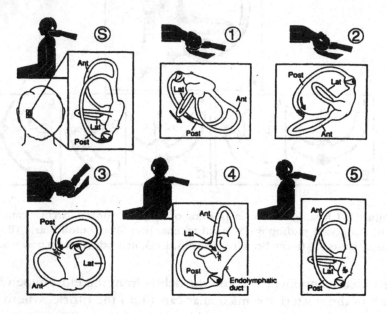

**Figure 9.3** The five stages of the particle-repositioning procedure for canalithiasis of left posterior semicircular canal, as described by Epley (1992) S=starting position. (Reproduced with permission.)

This procedure was first introduced by Epley in 1980 and a similar single-manoeuvre therapy was introduced by Semont, Freyss and Vitte in 1988. Reporting on the results of his five-position cycle for the treatment of BPPV, Epley (1992) emphasised the value of mastoid vibration at each stage of the manoeuvre, to ensure that all the debris is transferred to the most dependent part of the canal. He further reported that he medicated his patients before treatment, but subsequent workers have not found this necessary in most cases.

After the particle-repositioning procedure described by both Epley (1992) and Semont, Freyss and Vitte (1988), the patient is advised to remain in the upright position for at least 48 hours, even during the night. It may be helpful to provide a soft collar during this period to facilitate immobility. Epley (1992) further suggests that the patient should not sleep on the affected side for the next five days.

There is consensus that, if the initial treatment fails, the manoeuvre should be repeated. Approximately 10–20% of patients suffer a relapse or are not cured by the initial manoeuvre and some 10–20% of patients are reported to feel a persistent unsteadiness and/or disorientation, which may last for up to a week. There are no control studies to indicate whether mastoid vibration and the 48-hour period of maintaining a vertical position confer benefit in terms of outcome.

There are rare reports of patients becoming acutely vertiginous while particle-repositioning procedures are being performed and it has been suggested that this is the result of debris becoming obstructed in the posterior semicircular canal. This is accompanied by acute vertigo and vomiting and patients may require sedation and anti-emetics. It is for this reason that particle-repositioning procedures should be conducted in the presence of a medically qualified person. The correct management of this situation is the immediate 'reversal' of the five positions used in (for example) the Epley procedure, with mastoid vibration, which is hypothesised to bring about clearing of the canal.

In an unpublished series of patient studies reported by Shepard (personal communication), he has identified that the success rate of the particle-repositioning procedure is marginally lower in patients with additional evidence on caloric and/or electronystagmographic traces of peripheral vestibular dysfunction involving the horizontal semicircular canal. In this latter group, he identified a slightly greater number of patients requiring repeat particle-repositioning procedures to bring about resolution of their symptoms. Moreover, there may have been an additional requirement for physical exercise regimes to alleviate symptoms associated with the horizontal semicircular canal abnormality.

All workers adopting specific therapies for BPPV have reported excellent results (Table 9.11). Herdman et al. (1993) compared two different positional manoeuvres for treating BPPV and found a comparable cure rate of 70–90% with both. Rarely, patients present with prolonged, intractable BPPV, which is not corrected by the particle-repositioning procedure. In these cases, singular neurectomy (Gacek, 1978) or a canal plugging procedure (Parnes & McClure, 1991) may prove of value. The main complication of these procedures is the development of a sensorineural hearing loss, which has been reported in as many as 10% of patients.

Rarely, anterior and horizontal semicircular canal variants of BPPV may be observed (Table 9.12). The anterior canal variant may be treated successfully with the same particle repositioning treatment used for the posterior variant, whereas the horizontal canal variant is not cured by positional manoeuvres (Baloh, Jacobson & Honrubia, 1993).

**Table 9.11** Comparative efficacy of various treatments of BPPV

| Exercise protocol | No. of subjects | Improved or asymptomatic (%) | Duration of treatment |
|---|---|---|---|
| Brandt & Daroff (1980) | 67 | 98 | 3–14 days |
| Semont, Freyss & Vitte (1988) | 711 | 84 | 1 manoeuvre |
| Norré & Becker (1987) | 23 | 52 | 1 treatment |
| Habituation | 28 | 32 | 1 week |
| | | 100 | 6 weeks |
| Epley (1992) | 30 | 100 | multiple manoeuvres in one session |
| Herdman et al. (1993) | | | |
| modified Epley | 30 | 90 | 1 manoeuvre |
| Semont | 30 | 90 | 1 manoeuvre |

From Herdman (1994). Reproduced with permission.

**Table 9.12** Features of the three common varieties of BPPV

| | Posterior canal | Anterior canal | Horizontal canal |
|---|---|---|---|
| Relative incidence | 1.0 | 0.1 | 0.01 |
| Nystagmus direction | torsional up | torsional down | horizontal directional-changing |
| Inducing manoeuvre | sitting to head-hanging | sitting to head-hanging | supine to head-lateral |
| Duration (sec) | <30 | <30 | >30 |
| Latency (sec) | 5–15 | 5–15 | <3 |
| Fatigability | Yes | Yes | No |

From Baloh (1996). Reproduced with permission.

In conclusion, the value of physical exercise regimes and manoeuvres, although initially identified in the mid-1940s have, in the past 10 years, been shown to be the mainstay of rehabilitation in patients with dysequilibrium. Thus, patients who previously suffered protracted symptoms of dysequilibrium and moved *en bloc*, attempting to avoid any position which may precipitate their symptoms have been 'liberated' by understanding that active physical exercises which deliberately stimulate their symptoms, provide the means by which they recover. Moreover, the use of particle-repositioning procedures has revolutionised the management of BPPV. An understanding of the principles underlying physical exercise regimes and manoeuvres provides the patient with the confidence and determination to persevere in the face of what may initially seem to be a deterioration in their symptomatology and, together with a rehabilitation package, forms the cornerstone of good management of chronic vestibular symptoms.

# Chapter 10
# Physical exercise regimes – practical aspects

GAIL FOORD AND JON MARSDEN

## Introduction

This chapter describes the options for the physical treatment of unilateral peripheral vestibular disorders (PVD), alluding to bilateral and central disorders where relevant. The treatment of vertigo will be identified and the advantages and disadvantages of class instruction discussed. The associated disorders of balance and postural control, gaze stabilisation and eye–head coordination are considered. Finally, reference will be made to the treatment of benign paroxysmal positional vertigo (BPPV).

## Vertigo

Since the mid-1940s physiotherapists have taught Cawthorne Cooksey exercises (Cooksey, 1945) for the treatment of PVD. The exercises we perform today have been modified from the work of Dix (1974). These exercises are designed to restore balance and to facilitate the visual system and joint position sense to compensate for permanent vestibular dysfunction (Dix, 1974). At the National Hospital for Neurology and Neurosurgery, the adult neurological physiotherapy outpatient service is referred an average of 50 new patients each month for vestibular rehabilitation and most have a diagnosis of PVD. Approximately 80% of patients are treated in groups of 6–7 people. One physiotherapist and one physiotherapy assistant run the class jointly.

Cawthorne (1945) and Cooksey (1945) had patients exercise together in daily group sessions and Dix (1974) highlights this aspect of vestibular rehabilitation:

> It is a great advantage to group patients together for exercises. They encourage each other ... In the case of individual outpatients they should be accompanied by a friend or relative who also learns the exercises and can help the patient in practising them at home.

Wherever possible these exercises are taught in groups. This allows the physiotherapist more time to provide information to the patient. The skills mix of the physiotherapist and physiotherapy assistant utilises department staffing effectively and is cost-effective. In allocating specific gymnasium time to a class, it is possible to create an environment which is conducive to teaching exercises, i.e. spacious, quiet, safe and without distraction. The class has been shown to be a good forum for providing information and support (Freeman & Nairne, 1995) and it offers a chance for patients to discuss with the therapist and one another their symptoms and disabilities (Table 10.1). The principal disadvantage of class work is that patients with neck and back problems may find the exercises physically demanding and need individual instruction or the modification of the exercises.

Table 10.1 Symptoms and related disabilities of vestibular dysfunction

| Symptom | Disabilities |
| --- | --- |
| Vertigo and associated symptoms:<br>    vertigo<br>    disorientation<br>    nausea<br>    light/heavy-headed | Reduced mobility:<br>  e.g. difficulty using public transport<br>        difficulty walking in crowds<br>        difficulty travelling in cars<br>        dependent upon walking aid |
| Abnormalities of posture and gait:<br>    instability<br>    falls | Difficulty going out alone/<br>Housebound<br>Wheelchair bound |
| Musculo-skeletal symptoms:<br>    neck pain<br>    postural deformities | Reduced activities of daily living:<br>    difficulty performing domestic<br>    activities, e.g. ironing, washing<br>    difficulty shopping |
| Poor gaze stabilisation/eye–<br>head coordination<br>    blurred vision | Difficulty working<br>Limited leisure options |
| Psychological symptoms:<br>    fatigue<br>    anxiety<br>    low mood<br>    agoraphobia | Loss of confidence<br>Difficulty socialising<br>Inability to work |

Careful inclusion criteria are required as the class environment is generally not suitable for patients with severe hearing or visual impairments, severe physical disability or if a walking aid is required. If an interpreter is necessary an individual appointment is recommended. The class environment is also not suitable for patients with a psychiatric impairment, or when there is a marked illness behaviour component. Age is not a contraindication to class instruction. However, other medical conditions, such as hypertension, should be noted and the patient may be treated more appropriately on an individual basis.

### Aims and objectives of the class

The aim of the class is to provide a forum for the education of vestibular rehabilitation and a means of reducing the symptoms of vertigo by specific exercises (Figure 10.1). In order to meet these aims the class objectives are:

- Provision of background information on vestibular disturbance by means of introduction to the class (see teaching format below).
- Teaching of standard exercises based on the Cawthorne Cooksey regime.
- Provision of written information for review by doctor on follow-up.
- Provision of a named therapist and contact telephone number for ongoing enquiries.

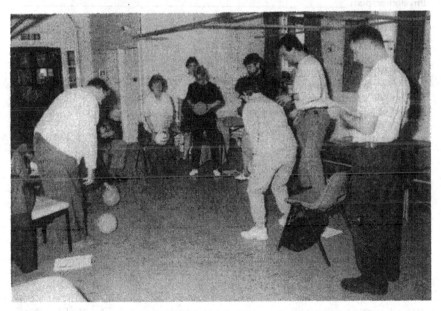

**Figure 10.1** Exercise class in progress.

### Teaching format

The following is the format used for teaching Cawthorne Cooksey exercises in both class and individual situations.

## Data collection sheet

As shown in Figure 10.2 this forms the basis of the therapist's assessment of the patient. It assists in indicating the factors which are likely to provoke the symptoms of vertigo. It is also the physiotherapist's record of the tailored exercise programme should the patient contact the department by telephone seeking further advice.

The patient is introduced to the anatomy of the structures involved in the disorder by use of a three-dimensional model of the ear, and the rationale behind the exercises and the scoring system is explained. In the group situation, patients are asked to share their symptoms and experiences of vertigo.

Vestibular Rehabilitation Physiotherapy Documentation
Cawthorne Cookesey

Patient name: _____ Male ☐                     Female ☐

Hospital No: _____ Telephone No: _____

Consultant:                               Diagnosis:

Age: _____ Address: _____

_____

Physiotherapist: _____

Signature: _____ Date: _____

1) What are your symptoms?
2) How long do they last?
3) How often do they occur?
4) When did they start?
5) Are they getting better or worse?
6) What precipitates your symptoms?
7) What makes them better?
8) What is your occupation?                      At work? ☐     Off work? ☐
9) Are you playing any sports?


To be completed by therapy staff.

10) Circle any exercises which aggravate

A. Eyes          1 2
B. Head          3 4 5 6
C. Trunk         7 8 9 10 11 12 13 14 15 16 17 18 19
D. Lying down    20 21 22 23 24 25 26 27

Cawthorne Cookesey management programme explained and given?   Yes ☐     No ☐

Nos. 1–9 are completed by the patient with assistance and discussion if necessary. No 10 is completed by the therapist/helper and is a record of which excersises provoked symptoms.


**Figure 10.2** The data collection sheet.

Exercises are performed and the symptoms provoked are rated. The exercises are demonstrated by either the physiotherapist or the physiotherapy assistant (see Figure 10.1 above).

Advice is given on how to continue and carry out the exercises during the subsequent months of the patient's rehabilitation. A telephone contact 'help line' number is provided.

Finally, relaxation and breathing exercises are performed as required.

It is the authors' experience that the ratio of staff to patients should be no fewer than 1:3.5. The skills mix of physiotherapist and physiotherapy assistant ensures that a therapist is available to answer questions which inevitably arise about the cause of the symptoms, the rationale of the exercises, and prognosis.

### Performance of the exercises

The exercise programme is tailored to an individual by means of a rating system (Figure 10.3). Patients are asked to perform the exercise five times and then to score their symptoms according to the following scale:

0 = no symptoms
1 = mild symptoms
2 = moderate symptoms
3 = severe symptoms.

This scale is subjective and relates to the individual's perceptions of his symptoms. All scored exercises are then marked with an asterisk and patients are instructed to work their way down the list of asterisked exercises as follows:

- Do only one exercise at a time.
- Do the exercise in three sets of five and repeat three times a day.
- Do not start on the next exercise until you no longer get any symptoms from the one you are doing (or if two weeks have passed by). (NB. This proviso was added to prevent patients getting 'stuck' on a single exercise.)
- Do only the exercises marked with an asterisk (*).

Patients are advised to perform the exercises until the symptoms are induced, but they are informed that they should not feel ill at the end of the session. However, patients are also told there may be a period when they may feel worse before they feel better (Herdman, 1994). A personal weekly rating chart is provided and patients

## Cawthorne Cooksey Exercises

| | | | | start date | one month | two months | three months |
|---|---|---|---|---|---|---|---|
| **Eyes** | Movements of your eye, keeping your head still | | | | | | |
| | 1) up & down, then side to side following your finger | 1 | | | | | |
| | 2) focusing on your finger moving 3 feet to 1 foot from your face. | 2 | | | | | |
| **Head** | | | | | | | |
| Eyes open | 3) bending forwards and backwards | 3 | | | | | |
| | 4) turning from side to side | 4 | | | | | |
| Eyes closed | 5) bending forwards and backwards | 5 | | | | | |
| | 6) turning from side to side | 6 | | | | | |
| **Trunk** | Eyes and head must follow the object | | | | | | |
| Eyes open | 7) from standing, bend forwards to pick up object from the floor and back up to standing | 7 | | | | | |
| | 8) from standing, bend forwards to pick up object from the floor, turn to left to place object behind, leave object, turn to right to pick up object, now place object back in front | 8 | | | | | |
| | 9) from standing, drop shoulders and head, sideways to left and then right | 9 | | | | | |
| | 10) from standing, reach with object up into the air to left then right | 10 | | | | | |
| | 11) from standing, pick object from floor and reach high into the air | 11 | | | | | |
| | 12) change sit to standing, turning one way sit down, stand up, turn opposite way, sit down | 12 | | | | | |
| | 13) turning on spot to left and right | 13 | | | | | |
| Eyes closed | 14) from standing, bend forward to touch floor and back to standing | 14 | | | | | |
| | 15) from standing, bend forwards to touch floor, turn to left touch chair behind, turn to right to touch chair, back to the front | 15 | | | | | |
| | 16) from standing, drop shoulders and head, sideways to left and then right | 16 | | | | | |
| | 17) from standing, touch floor, reach high into the air | 17 | | | | | |
| | 18) change sit to standing, turning one way sit down, stand up, turn opposite way sit down | 18 | | | | | |
| | 19) turning on spot to left and right | 19 | | | | | |
| **Lying down** | If possible do not use a pillow | | | | | | |
| Eye open | 20) rolling head from side to side | 20 | | | | | |
| | 21) rolling whole body from side to side | 21 | | | | | |
| | 22) sitting up straight forwards | 22 | | | | | |
| | 23) from lying, roll onto your side, sit up over edge of bed, lie down on opposite side and roll onto your back | 23 | | | | | |
| Eyes closed | 24) rolling head from side to side | 24 | | | | | |
| | 25) rolling whole body from side to side | 25 | | | | | |
| | 26) sitting up straight forwards | 26 | | | | | |
| | 27) from lying, roll onto your side, sit up over edge of the bed, lie down on opposite side and roll onto your back | 27 | | | | | |

NB. All exercises to be done at a moderate speed. Any of these exercises may require supervision to ensure sa

**Figure 10.3** The revised exercise programme rating system.

are encouraged to identify which exercise they are performing and to rate it either once a week or when they progress to their next exercise. In this way, patients can monitor their own progress by noting the severity of symptoms on the scale noted above.

Finally, all patients receive the name of a physiotherapist and a 'help line' telephone number, which they may use if they are at all worried or have any questions. General enquiries are made when patients need to discuss the effect of an exercise or activity on their symptoms or if they are not progressing. Between 5 and 10% of all patients telephone for further guidance and support from the physiotherapist.

In both class and individual instruction all patients are seen once at the Physiotherapy Department and are followed up by their neuro-otologist within 1–3 months. They are instructed to take their exercise programme and personal weekly rating chart with them to their follow-up appointment. This assists both patient and doctor with the assessment of progress. In some cases (for example, those with very severe symptoms who could not complete the exercises) patients are given an extra individual appointment for further advice. Smith-Wheelock, Shepard and Telian (1991) suggest that regular outpatient physiotherapy visits may be indicated for patients with a high probability of non-compliance, those who lack the cognitive abilities to manage the programme, and those who inappropriately persist in 'believing that there is some sort of medication or surgery available to "cure" their symptoms'. Patients who require other treatment modalities as part of their rehabilitation will be seen as often as indicated by the condition and their progress.

It was shown by Freeman and Nairne (1995) that the class situation provided an effective forum for giving information, support and a means of rehabilitation to people with vestibular dysfunction. It proved effective both in terms of cost and use of therapist time and had the additional support of other group members. Comments received by Freeman and Nairn (1995) from patients included:

- "Very informative and quite a relief that there are other people who suffer and that it is not all in my mind."
- "Very helpful and reassuring. I like being with others in my condition."
- "The class helped to reassure me that I can help myself better and not depend on medication for the rest of my life."
- "I wish I had this class 10 months ago when I first got my illness."

In physiotherapy we receive anecdotal reports from both the Neuro-Otology Department and patients that the exercises are effective. A pilot study has shown that this regime improves movement-induced vertigo in patients with PVD (Savundra et al., 1993).

and a joint study is planned to evaluate the outcome of this programme in detail. It must also be stated that one of the reasons for the success of the programme is the team of professionals involved, as emphasised by Shepard and Telian (1995).

In summary, the principal physiotherapy treatment modality for the rehabilitation of PVD is the modified Cawthorne Cooksey programme. Where any modifications have been made to the exercise programme described by Dix (1974), it has been with the aim of simplifying the programme and making it more manageable for patients to perform unassisted and within the limits of safety. Strong emphasis is placed on cardiovascular fitness, return to a normal lifestyle and sport as part of rehabilitation, as elements of these aid in the compensation process.

A similar approach was advocated by Norré (cited by Herdman, Borello-France & Whitney, 1994) which he referred to as 'habituation training'. He developed a series of 19 vertigo-provoking manoeuvres from activities of daily living and asked each patient to indicate how often they performed each activity on a scale of 0–6, i.e. 'Never' to 'Very often'. Norré believed patients avoided such movements in an attempt to decrease their chance of precipitating an episode of vertigo and advocated that the use of specific habituation exercises could therefore help promote adaptation of the vestibular system (Herdman, Borello-France & Whitney, 1994).

## Balance and postural control

To be able to balance successfully and adapt to a wide variety of constantly changing environmental and internal conditions requires a normal postural control system (Massion, 1994). This must be assessed in its entirety. The postural control system ultimately controls the musculoskeletal system (Horak & Shupert, 1994; Keshner, 1994; Shumway-Cook & Woollacott, 1995a).

### Musculoskeletal impairments

Impairments, such as limb or truncal weakness, decreased joint range of motion or pain, are common especially in the elderly population (Horak, Shupert & Mirka, 1989). These will directly influence the ability to balance and can often be readily improved with physiotherapy intervention (Shumway-Cook & Woollacott, 1995b). Of particular note is neck stiffness/pain, which often occurs with vestibular disorders (Shumway-Cook & Horak, 1990). Neck immobility is thought to arise in an attempt (often subconscious) either to decrease the unpleasant feelings of vertigo and/or oscillopsia which are induced by head motion or to enhance the cervico-ocular reflex and so aid gaze stabilisation (Horak & Shupert, 1994). Neck stiffness or pain may prevent patients to reproduce their symptoms of vertigo and in the long term will prevent or slow any compensatory processes (Borello-France, Whitney & Herdman, 1994). With vestibular rehabilitation this may improve sponta-neously, but on occasions will require a specialist musculoskeletal physiotherapist.

### Sensory impairments

Normal postural control under varying conditions relies on vestibu-lar, visual and somatosensory sensation (Shumway-Cook & Woolla-cott, 1995a). Following a vestibular lesion, we need to consider whether the deficit is a unilateral or bilateral peripheral disorder, whether the patient over-relies on one particular sensory input, i.e. vision or somatosensory sensation, and whether there is any other sensory impairment present.

#### Unilateral versus bilateral peripheral deficits

In the case of a complete bilateral deficit, under certain conditions the patient will always be unbalanced, for example, when illumina-tion is poor and somatosensory cues are unreliable i.e., walking on a slope or in the dark. Physiotherapy must be directed at teaching patients why and when they will experience imbalance and strate-gies to avoid this, such as switching the lights on before getting out of bed. The patient with bilateral vestibular deficit, unlike most patients with a unilateral disorder, may require a walking aid, espe-cially in the early stages (Herdman, 1994) but care should be taken that the patient does not become dependent on such an aid.

Studies on patients with bilateral vestibular hypofunction demonstrate that vestibular rehabilitation can be effective on this patient group (Gill-Body & Krebs, 1994). In a double-blind randomised clinical trial, patients who performed vestibular reha-bilitation significantly improved in terms of the frequency and severity of their symptoms and stability, as indicated by a decrease in the time spent in the double stance phase of gait (Krebs et al., 1993). Other authors have found similar improvements in balance and gait, although they found no improvement in oscillopsia (Shep-ard & Telian, 1995).

For peripheral vestibular disorders one needs to assess whether use is being made of remaining vestibular input or whether there is over-reliance on a particular sensory modality.

### Over-reliance on a given sensory modality

Immediately following an acute episode, PVD patients frequently over-rely on input from their visual system, ignoring available input from their vestibular and somatosensory systems. Sometimes a moving visual scene (for example, trucks passing in front of the patient in the street) can be misinterpreted as self-motion and 'corrective' postural adjustments are produced which in the circumstances can cause postural instability (Horak & Shupert, 1994; Bronstein, 1995).

When devising an exercise programme which addresses this problem, the physiotherapist must assess the sensation upon which the patient is relying. This may be evident following subjective assessment but may require more specific testing.

The *Clinical Test for Sensory Integration in Balance* (CTSIB) was developed from laboratory posturography tests (Norré, 1994; Di Fabio, 1995; Furman, 1995). The test examines the patient's body sway under a variety of altered sensory conditions (Shumway-Cook & Horak, 1986). If patients rely more on vision, for example, they will increase their body sway when vision is distorted or absent even though some vestibular or somatosensory sensation may be present (Shumway-Cook & Horak, 1989). If the patient is found to rely disproportionately on one sensory input specific treatments can be devised. For example, if the patient over-relies on vision, tasks can be devised whereby the patient must balance during functional activities with reduced or distorted visual input but good somatosensory input (for example, in bare feet) at first.

In order to teach patients to rely on their remaining vestibular sensation, gradual reduction of visual and sensory cues is needed. There is no fixed formula for this training. All vestibular rehabilitation is aimed at improving the patient's functional difficulties and the therapist must assess which tasks the patient finds difficult, determine why and then develop treatment programmes aimed at alleviating them (Shumway-Cook & Horak, 1989; Horak, 1994).

### The importance of vision and somatosensation

If the patient with a peripheral vestibular disorder has a concomitant somatosensory or visual impairment this will affect the ability to compensate for the vestibular dysfunction (Smith & Curthoys, 1989) and may require the teaching of protective strategies.

### Impairments in movement strategies

The central components of the postural control system involve many inter-related systems (Pompeiano, 1994). Lesions to these systems which are implicated in the compensation process and in adaptation to altering conditions can affect the prognosis for recovery. For example, patients with persisting imbalance and vertigo may have a cerebellar lesion as well as a peripheral vestibular disorder (Rudge & Chambers, 1982; Curthoys & Halmagyi, 1995).

Correct processing of incoming sensory information allows a person to develop a correct perceptual awareness of their orientation in space, their limits of stability and allows them to programme movement strategies which are relevant to the present and forthcoming environmental conditions (Horak & Shupert, 1994). There are three main postural strategies needed to recover balance in standing: an ankle strategy; a hip strategy; and a stepping strategy. Postural movement strategies need to be assessed under different task conditions, for example, during self-initiated postural sway, following a perturbation, or in anticipation of a voluntary movement (Shumway-Cook et al., 1996).

Vestibular input seems to be needed to perform a hip strategy, which is used when balancing on a small base of support, a compliant surface or when recovering equilibrium when the person is balancing at the limits of stability (Horak & Shupert, 1994). Following total bilateral vestibular loss, the patient cannot use a hip strategy and can get 'stuck' on an ankle strategy, which relies more on somatosensory input. With irritative vestibular lesions, however, the patient may use excessive hip and trunk movement during balancing (Black et al., 1988; Shupert, Horak & Black, 1994). The latter can have severe practical implications. The hip strategy relies on the transmission of shear forces to the ground caused by large proximal movement of the trunk and hips. In cases where the frictional forces between the ground and the person are poor (such as standing on a slippery surface), the use of a hip strategy could cause a fall as there is insufficient frictional force present (Shumway-Cook & Horak, 1986).

It has been suggested that patients can be retrained to use a given strategy which they do not automatically utilise. The patient is taught to perform a given stategy during self-initiated sway, tasks involving voluntary limb movements and in response to perturbations (Shumway-Cook & Horak, 1986; Shumway-Cook et al., 1996).

**Impairments of the perception of vertical and stability limits**

Frequently, patients with severe sensory loss or a central vestibular disorder (for example, Wallenburg's syndrome) can have poor perception of their vertical mid-line, visual vertical and their stability limits (Dieterich & Brandt, 1990; Brandt & Dieterich, 1993). During balance retraining which includes varying sensory conditions and varying movement strategies, verbal, visual and biofeedback about a patient's orientation may be helpful in teaching them to have a normal perception of body orientation in space (Shumway-Cook & Horak, 1990).

# Gaze stabilisation and eye–head coordination

The vestibular system is vital for normal gaze stabilisation and eye–head coordination (Kasai & Zee, 1978; Guitton, 1992; Roucoux, 1992).

### Gaze stabilisation

Following bilateral vestibular deficit the absence of the vestibulo-ocular reflex (VOR) and therefore gaze stabilisation is manifested by oscillopsia with head movements or walking (Takahashi et al., 1988; Grossman & Leigh, 1990). Patients can compensate for poor gaze stabilisation by enhancing their cervico-ocular reflex, performing compensatory eye movements and by changing their perception of the oscillopsia (Leigh, 1994). After a unilateral disorder the VOR will underfunction, i.e. have a low gain, and recalibration of the VOR gain is required.

Patients can be clinically assessed as to whether they can stabilise their gaze during voluntary and involuntary head or head/trunk movement while sitting, standing or walking. Any corrective saccades and any subjective feelings of blurring or unstable vision are noted. Exercises aimed at teaching patients to stabilise their gaze in relevant situations can be prescribed (Lerner, Washko & Gilbert, 1991; Herdman et al., 1994). The exercises are similar for the bilateral and unilateral vestibular disorders, although the methods of compensation may differ (Herdman, 1994). For example, the patient could perform vertical and horizontal head movements while fixating a visual target at arm's length or across the room (Herdman, 1995). A target with words on, such as a business card, could be used and patients would move their head gently back and forth for a minute while keeping the target in focus (Herdman, Borello-France & Whitney, 1994).

One study examined gaze stabilisation exercises, with head movement performed by patients in the acute stages following removal of an acoustic neuroma. The exercises were performed for one minute each in sitting and standing positions, five times a day, for a total of 20 minutes. Control subjects performed smooth pursuit eye movements with no head movement post-operatively for the same amount of time as the 'vestibular adaptation' group. There was a significantly greater percentage of patients with a normal VOR as assessed clinically six days post-operatively in the 'vestibular adaptation group' as compared with the controls. The 'vestibular adaptation' group also significantly improved in their subjective reports of dysequilibrium and postural stability as assessed by use of posturography and clincal gait analysis (Herdman, 1995).

### Eye–head coordination

First, saccadic and pursuit eye movements with the head stationary are assessed. Then, the ability to locate targets in near and far periphery, using coordinated eye–head–trunk movements, is evaluated. The movement coordination can be scored subjectively as intact, impaired or unable (Shumway-Cook & Woollacott, 1995c; Shumway-Cook et al., 1996).

Following assessment in a variety of positions and tasks eye–head coordination exercises can be prescribed which are, once again, patient-specific. As the pattern of eye–head coordination alters when reaching and grasping with the arm, functional tasks involving eye–head–hand coordination should also be performed (Carnahan, 1992; Vercher et al., 1994), for example, foveating and reaching for cups close to and then further away from the patient in both the horizontal and vertical planes.

Although Cawthorne Cooksey exercises do involve some degree of eye–head coordination and gaze stabilisation these functions are not usually assessed formally or specifically treated in isolation by physiotherapists in the UK. This is an area which should be developed in close liaison with neuro-otologists to improve clinical assessment and treatment.

## Effectiveness of vestibular rehabilitation

Studies examining the effectiveness of a generic exercise programme, such as the Cawthorne Cooksey exercises previously described, and a customised exercise programme which is individually designed for the patient, have been encouraging.

Recently, a clinical trial compared the effects of modified Cawthorne Cooksey exercises with the effects of an anti-vertigo drug (betahistine mesylate) in patients with acute unilateral vestibular disturbances not due to BPPV or Ménière's disease (Fujino et al., 1996). The signs and symptoms of the two patient groups were not significantly different before any treatment. The vestibular training group performed a block of modified Cawthorne Cooksey exercises for 15 minutes three times a day. Compared with the patients who did not exercise and took the anti-vertigo medication, the vestibular training group showed a significant improvement in the symptoms of vertigo. The vestibular training group also demonstrated a significantly greater improvement in their impairments in balance, as measured by the sharpened Romberg's test and spontaneous and positional nystagmus, as assessed clinically by use of Frenzel's spectacles and during the Hallpike–Dix manoeuvre.

The effectiveness of individually customised vestibular rehabilitation has also been evaluated experimentally. Improvement in subjective symptoms of dizziness and imbalance and in objective measures of balance, gait and spontaneous or postural nystagmus have been reported. Types of conditions studied include, acute (Herdman, 1995) and chronic (Shepard et al., 1993), unilateral (Horak, 1994) and bilateral (Krebs et al., 1993), peripheral disorders and central vestibular disorders (Shepard & Telian, 1995). One follow-up study by questionnaire demonstrated that although most patients had some persisting symptoms of imbalance and motion-provoked dizziness, improvement with rehabilitation was generally maintained for the 12–36 month period of the study (Smith-Wheelock, Shepard & Telian, 1991).

It is a general consensus that although certain conditions, such as central disorders, head injury and patients with severe persistent disability have a worse prognosis in terms of time taken to recover and eventual improvement in disability and imbalance, this should not preclude rehabilitation (Shepard et al., 1993).

To date there have been no papers written comparing the two types of vestibular rehabilitation, generic and customised treatment, although a three-year prospective randomised trial is being performed in Michigan by Shepard and colleagues (Shepard et al., 1993).

# Benign paroxysmal positional vertigo

Brandt and Daroff (1980) devised a sequence of repetitive positioning for the treatment of benign paroxysmal positional vertigo (BPPV). The presumed mechanism of the basis of these exercises is the loosening and ultimate dispersion of degenerated otolithic particles from the cupula of the posterior semicircular canal (Brandt & Daroff, 1980).

Patients undergo a series of repetitive positionings. From the sitting position the patient lies down sideways to adopt the position which brings on the vertigo. Once the symptoms subside the patient sits up and then lies down on the opposite side (see Figure 9.2). This sequence of positions is continued until the patient no longer has the symptoms. Each series of exercises is performed 3–4 times per day until the patient has two consecutive vertigo-free days. Brandt–Daroff exercises have now been largely superseded by the canalith repositioning procedure – 'Epley manoeuvre' (Epley, 1992). This is designed to treat BPPV through induced 'out-migration' of free-moving pathological densities in the endolymph of the semicircular canal, using timed head manoeuvres and applied vibration. This procedure is generally performed by a doctor in the neuro-otology clinic (Chapter 9). The comparative efficacy of various BPPV treatments has been studied by Girardi, Horst and Konrad (1996). The Brandt–Daroff exercise and the Epley manoeuvre have both been shown to be highly effective for the treatment of BPPV.

In conclusion, physical exercise regimes are the mainstay of vestibular rehabilitation. They appear to be most effective when directed by an experienced and specialised department. Important components include a positive approach, adequate diagnostic facilities and the introduction of an appropriate rehabilitation programme for each patient. Adequate and available practical support for a self-administered exercise programme is necessary. Monitoring of progress, leading to a return to a normal lifestyle, with discharge from the clinic, being the ultimate goal.

# Chapter 11
# Relaxation for patients with peripheral vestibular disorders

RACHEL FABER RUTLEY

## Introduction

This chapter aims to explain the rationale for the use of relaxation techniques with patients who have a peripheral vestibular disorder (PVD) and show its context as part of a vestibular rehabilitation programme. It has been shown that a significant number of patients with PVD have a psychological component to their disability (Eagger et al., 1991). Relaxation can be a useful technique in reducing the effects of stress and anxiety, which are sometimes experienced as a secondary component of a patient's disequilibrium, thus enabling a more effective recovery through the use of Cawthorne Cooksey exercises.

## Secondary symptoms of vertigo

In addition to the commonly accepted symptoms of dizziness, blurred vision, nausea and unsteadiness, patients with vertigo have also frequently been noted to present with the seondary symptoms of neck pain, increased muscle tension, fatigue, anxiety and low mood (Brown, 1990; Shumway-Cook & Horak, 1990; Smith, 1990). There are indications that these secondary symptoms may be linked to prior psychiatric disturbances or even psychiatric disorders, which develop following the onset of their vertigo. A study by Eagger et al. (1991) investigated the pyschiatric morbidity of patients with PVD. In 54 patients who had PVD and were interviewed and tested in detail, 25% had experience of psychiatric illness prior to the onset of their neuro-otological symptoms. The most common diagnoses were generalised anxiety disorders and major depression. Sixty-five per cent of the patients were also classified as experiencing psychiatric illness for some period since the onset of their symptoms. In nearly two-thirds of these cases this had occurred during the first six months after onset of their neuro-otological problems. Most commonly, the symptoms were panic disorder, with or without agoraphobia, and major depressive illness. The agoraphobia was linked to problems with self-perception and social interaction, such as being self-conscious of appearing drunk or losing balance while walking. Yardley (1994) suggests that these types of panic reactions may originate with autonomic symptoms, which originally formed part of the syndrome of spontaneous acute vertigo.

The presence of any type of psychiatric disorder, ranging from stress and depression to generalised anxiety disorders and panic attacks, may contribute to the development of the secondary symptoms of vertigo as described above. The study by Eagger et al. (1991) also suggested that recovery is likely to be slower once the symptoms have become more chronic. This highlights the need to diagnose PVD as early as possible and apply effective and appropriate treatment strategies to prevent the development of secondary symptoms related to stress and generalised anxiety disorders, which may delay or even preclude any spontaneous recovery.

The secondary symptoms of vertigo described can be likened to the symptoms of stress. The body's stress response occurs when it responds to changes in the external or internal environment, when these changes are perceived as placing a demand upon the system. Under conditions of stress, an individual's neuro-otological symptoms of vertigo and dizziness are likely to be exacerbated.

## Components of the stress response

For the stress response to be triggered a demand must be placed on the system. In the context of the dizzy patient the stressor is likely to be the ongoing dysequilibrium with its associated symptoms and the negative effect which this has on his usual function. The patient's perception of the stressor is also significant. One person may easily ignore or brush off minor symptoms of dizziness, whereas for another the equivalent level of symptoms may be experienced acutely and cause significantly greater levels of anxiety. The individual's response will be further affected by the various psychological and social influences on their personality. Together, the psychological and physical responses of the body to stress cause a build-up of energy to respond to the demands of the stressor. This phenomenon is a normal part of most people's everyday life and in some degree helps them to cope with the activities which they do. In fact, some degree of stress and tension is often considered necessary for normal adaptation and adjustment; it can be a motivator and help with the anticipation of deadlines and the achievement of events. For some, stress is perceived as an essential part of life and provides a sense of excitement, successful coping, satisfaction and fulfilment in all aspects of their lives.

Unfortunately, stress does not always produce such favourable outcomes. Ongoing unwanted stress or anxiety can become chronic and uncontrollable. This situation has been described by Johnson, Manchester and Sugden (1985) as causing a pathological anxiety, where the stress serves no useful purpose to the individual. The feeling induced is a type of fear or apprehension and leads to associated physiological changes. The ensuing state can be closely related to the well-known 'fight or flight' reaction.

## Reactions of the body to stress or anxiety

Some specific reactions have been noted to be associated with fear, stress and anxiety. According to Cannon (1953) systemically these reactions include:

- *A heightened awareness of external stimuli* as a preparation for defence of the perceived danger or stressor. In the context of the dizzy patient, this is the need to cope with the constant dysequilibrium and anxiety experienced.
- *Hormonal release from the pituitary gland.*
- *Generalised signals to the body from the nervous system* producing a system ready for any action and necessary responses.
- *Release of adrenaline and noradrenaline* from the adrenal glands.

These systemic reactions produce specific symptoms in a stressed or anxious person, which include:

- *Mental alertness* with a heightened awareness of all stimuli, the senses being over-reactive to the inputs which they receive. This causes some people to appear constantly on edge or nervous.
- *Hyperventilation.* This causes disorientation and confusion in a dizzy patient (Yardley, 1994). Theunissen, Huygen and Folering (1986) highlighted the control of hyperventilation as a significant component of vestibular dysfunction rehabilitation and the psychological adaptation which occurs in the recovering patient (Chapter 8).
- *Tachycardia* with increased blood pressure.

- *The release of sugars and fatty acids* into the bloodstream from the liver to supply rapid energy to the muscles.
- *Reduced immune responses* – this occurs in the short term to allow a large response elsewhere in the body. However, over an extended period this can become harmful.
- *Increased sweating* to cool the body.
- *Increased bloodflow to the muscles*, with tense muscle fibres, ready for action.

Additional chronic symptoms include:

- Headaches.
- Fatigue.
- Gastrointestinal disorders.
- Skin rashes.
- Allergy problems.
- Altered sleep patterns

People who experience abnormal anxiety are also likely to have certain psychological symptoms. These include apprehension, diffuse fear, and an inability to concentrate and panic (Johnson, Manchester & Sugden, 1985). The presence of these factors is unlikely to encourage patients to persevere with their Cawthorne Cooksey exercises, which deliberately provoke their symptoms, pushing themselves to the limit and potentially increase their stress and anxiety. These symptoms can be undeniably disturbing and, as Barber and Leigh (1988) suggest, the avoidance of head positions which provoke the symptoms of vertigo is a common factor in patients with ongoing vertigo. Over the extended period of time that their symptoms have occurred patients may have an upwardly spiralling increase of apprehension, fear and panic, which reinforces their secondary symptoms of chronic anxiety and so their primary symptoms of dysequilibrium.

Thus, to summarise, if a dizzy patient is of a particularly anxious nature or has a predisposing relevant psychiatric disorder, he or she may enter a chronic downward spiral of symptom avoidance, with the fear of any provocation leading to increased stress and tension and potential pathological anxiety. This will induce an increase in symptoms and an exaggerated avoidance of any advantageous compensatory movements, causing further deterioration. This is the scenario of chronic vertigo and chronic disability.

In order to break this spiralling deterioration in dizziness, relaxation can be a valuable adjunct to the use of physical exercise regimes to increase compliance in susceptible patients and help them cope with any potential increase in anxiety. In a study carried out at the National Hospital for Neurology and Neurosurgery (Savundra et al., 1993) it was shown that relaxation alone did have a significant effect in reducing the symptoms of vertigo in both PVD patients and patients with benign paroxysmal positional vertigo (BPPV). This effect was not so great as that achieved through the use of Cawthorne Cooksey exercises alone and, accordingly, relaxation is used as a component of the latter programme.

Relaxation is a way of producing a quiet body and calm mind. This physical and mental unwinding has been termed the 'relaxation response' by Benson (1975). Relaxation is presented as an antidote to the anxiety stage or stress response and can be taught to patients and incorporated as part of a self-administered programme.

## The relaxation response

As with the considerable effects shown to occur with the stress response, relaxation also has certain specific effects on the body (Benson, 1975):

- The hypothalamus of the brain causes the pituitary gland and the involuntary nervous system to bring about relaxation change and brain waves become slower.
- Breathing slows or becomes shallower as less oxygen is required.
- The heart rate decreases and the blood pressure drops.
- The adrenal glands no longer produce stress hormones and their presence in the blood stream decreases rapidly.
- Sweating decreases markedly.
- Lower electrical activity occurs in the muscles demonstrating a marked decrease in muscle tension.

One of the most easily measured physiological changes which occurs during deep relaxation is the alteration in the electrical activity occurring in the brain. As stated above, the hypothalamus influences the pituitary gland and involuntary nervous system leading to slower brain waves. In deep sleep, delta waves with a frequency of 1–4 cycles per second are present. In drowsy sleep, delta waves at a frequency of 4–7 cycles per second are present, appear to occur on the brink of sleep or unconsciousness and may be associated with dreamlike hypnagogic imagery. In the active brain state when a person should be awake, alert and thinking, beta waves with a frequency of 13 cycles per second are present. Between these last two frequencies alpha waves occur, with a frequency of 8–12 cycles per second. These usually occur when a person is awake but allows their mind to 'let go', a situation which can be more easily achieved for some than others within a normal population! An increased presence of alpha waves shows the achievement of reduced logical thought and a peaceful, tranquil state of mind. It is the dominance of this type of brain waves which occurs during successful relaxation (Sterman, 1974).

# Methods of relaxation

There are many ways of achieving a relaxation response. In this text ,a sample of the physically mediated methods of relaxation will be outlined. There is some thought that more physically mediated methods of relaxation can achieve an increased physical effect on the body during relaxation (Health Media & Education Centre, 1987). Since the aim with a dizzy patient is to reduce the anxiety caused by ongoing physical symptoms, the use of these methods would seem logical. However, this factor should not be over-emphasised since all relaxation methods include a strong psychological component which cannot be discounted.

### Progressive relaxation training

This was first proposed by Jacobson in the 1930s (Keable, 1989). It was a forerunner to many other modern relaxation methods and involves the development of advanced muscular skills. Progressive relaxation training aims to recognise and release minute amounts of tension within the muscles. It requires a long training period with daily sessions of hours and includes movements involving flexion and extension practised for all muscle groups.

Jacobson proposed that relaxation mediated by this method was caused by a powerful feedback loop linking the skeletal muscles and the brain. He suggested that the mind has the power to affect the state of the muscles and, in turn, by altering the state of the muscles, the mind can also be affected.

There are some problems with this method. It is a somewhat technical and skilled method and involves a great deal of time and commitment on the part of the patient and the tutor. Since the skill level required by the patient is relatively high, it is possible that patient compliance may be poor. In our modern healthcare environment, this method may also be costly.

### Biofeedback

Miller (1969) was one of the first proponents of this method. Biofeedback relies on the use of electrical equipment to give continuous biological information relating to arousal levels in the body.

Possible useful sources of information range from the heart rate, skin conductance or resistance, brain wave activity, blood pressure, skin temperature, and voluntary muscle tension in selected sites. Feedback can be given via auditory bleeps, and visually, by flashing lights and meter readings. The patient is taught to relate changes in the readings or noise levels to their voluntary release of tension. Studies have shown that individuals can learn to control autonomic responses, as well as voluntary muscle activity via this technique (Keable, 1989). In theory, the improved control achieved through biofeedback is mediated by 'operant conditioning', where a subject is given information which is not normally consciously acknowledged in order to develop a relaxed state in their muscles. However, as with most of the other methods of relaxation, the exact mechanism of this technique is unclear.

There are several criticisms of biofeedback. It is questionable as to whether the changes which are brought about are by cognitive manipulation or, in fact, by the purposeful skeletal muscular changes which also occur. It may also be the case that the peaceful thoughts required to concentrate on the equipment used in this approach may actually cause the change which is observed rather than the direct effect of the sophisticated equipment connected to the patient. It is also unclear whether the response observed through biofeedback is actually transferable to the patient's daily function or merely achieved during the treatment session. (In fairness, this criticism could be levied at most techniques of relaxation.) The cost associated with early equipment used for biofeedback and its cumbersome size are other frequently cited criticisms, although these factors have improved with modern machines becoming more technically sophisticated and competitive. One other consideration of note is that individuals respond differently with respect to which physiological systems react most to the stress which they experience. It may therefore be difficult to standardise and study the effects of biofeedback. It is possible that ordinary relaxation may be as or even more effective than biofeedback itself (Silver & Blanchard, 1978). Despite these shortcomings, biofeedback can be a useful technique to demonstrate the possible effects of relaxation to patients.

## Simple physiological relaxation

This approach was developed by Mitchell (1977), a physiotherapist. It involves the precise movements of the agonist muscle groups rather than the action of the opposing antagonist muscle groups. It is based on the principle of reciprocal innervation relating to voluntary muscles. The agonist muscle group moves the body part into a relaxed position, thus demanding that the antagonist muscle group relaxes to allow the movement to occur and the new position to be established. Therefore, as one muscle group moves, its opposer 'switches off' to accommodate the change of position. Other components of this method include:

- The involvement of relaxed breathing.
- Mental registering of the new position of ease produced by the agonist muscle groups.
- Use of individually selected distracting cognitive sequencing, for example, repetition of a poem while the person is actually performing the relaxation.
- Instruction to ignore unpleasant thoughts throughout the relaxation.

This technique stresses the role of joint proprioceptors and skin pressure receptors, which have pathways to higher brain centres unlike the muscle receptors. The person becomes trained to recognise the relaxed position and learns key positions and movements which can be used to initiate generalised relaxation during activity.

Little investigation has been done into these claims and again, as with other techniques, most of the evidence for its effectiveness over another method is anecdotal. It is a relatively cost-effective technique, requiring a simple session of instruction, often reinforced by the independent use of audio tapes by the patient.

**Contrast relaxation**

This technique was developed from Jacobson's Progressive Relaxation Training method by Wolpe in 1958 (Keable, 1989). It was originally a component for his systematic desensitisation procedure for the treatment of specific phobias. As a relaxation technique, it involves tensing and releasing exercises of the antagonist muscle groups. It is a quick and convenient technique, being taught in a single session. Contrast relaxation is based on the theory that a physiological relaxation will occur following maximal contraction in a muscle group. The subject is instructed to mentally register the new position of ease created by this release of tension.

As with Mitchell's simple physiological relaxation, there has been little investigation into the claims of contrast relaxation. It appears to be useful in giving the patient a good initial perception of the release of muscle tension and the feelings associated with it. Further research is needed into the overall effects of relaxation and its ability to reduce the amount of stress or anxiety experienced by patients in their daily lives.

## Current practice

As stated before, relaxation is not necessary or appropriate for every patient as part of a vestibular rehabilitation programme. It is used selectively with those patients who are known to have a significant psychological component to their condition to improve their compliance with the performance of Cawthorne Cooksey exercises. It may also be used where a clinician or therapist considers it would be beneficial following examination of a patient in whom a higher anxiety level is detected.

At the National Hospital for Neurology and Neurosurgery, patients are taught a form of contrast relaxation. They are instructed in the technique in an individual treatment session, initially supine, then being taught progressively to move into sitting and later standing positions, as they become more adept with the technique. Patients are taught to tense the antagonist muscle groups in turn and note the release of tension which occurs. The facial muscles are included in this process. Throughout the procedure, breathing exercises are used to reduce the breathing and keep the mind calm. Patients are instructed to do this daily in the positions described above, for a maximum of 20–30 minutes.

It is important to include an educational element in the teaching of relaxation. The patient should be informed that they will find the Cawthorne Cooksey exercises more beneficial when performed in conjunction with a relaxation programme. Increasing patients' knowledge of their condition and the programme they have learned is a useful reinforcement and aims to enhance their sense of personal control and expectation of a successful recovery.

## Summary

Relaxation can be a useful component of a rehabilitation programme for some patients with a peripheral vestibular disorder. When utilised effectively by an appropriate patient, it can increase the ability to cope with symptoms and the additional exposure required by the performance of daily Cawthorne Cooksey exercises. As an antidote to the secondary symptoms of stress often seen in dizzy patients, relaxation can also help prevent the downward spiralling of symptoms and encourage recovery instead of the typical chronic scenario frequently encountered in specialist departments.

# Chapter 12
# Outcome measures in vestibular rehabilitation

PETER SAVUNDRA

## Background

High-quality care should be reflected by good outcomes and these will attract the referrals and the funding which allow the development of service provision and clinical research. However, even to maintain current service levels, outcome measures have become important – with many purchasers now pushing to include outcome criteria in their contracts, as a means of assessing effectiveness. Indeed, some are placing as great an emphasis on this as on audits, which simply assess the process of care. This approach is based on the premise that medicine should be evidence-based (Evidence-based Medicine Working Group, 1992; Rosenberg & Donald, 1995) and it is, of course, entirely justifiable that clinical (and purchasing) decisions should be based on the best available scientific evidence.

The publication *Supporting Research and Development in the NHS* (Research and Development Task Force, 1994) mapped out for the first time the comprehensive strategy required for the funding of research in the NHS, and its provisions highlight the requirement to formalise the outcome concepts held by all those involved in clinical care.

It is generally agreed that randomised, prospective, double-blind controlled studies are the 'gold standard' to establish the effectiveness of a treatment regime (Cochrane, 1972). Alternative study models are bedevilled by the problems of differences in case-mix (Green et al., 1990) and uncontrolled studies fail to define the extent of spontaneous recovery or recovery due to a placebo effect. 'N of 1' studies, which have a role in drug treatment, have no place in rehabilitation medicine. Placebo-controlled studies are essential to define the effectiveness of a treatment regime and comparative trials are required to determine the efficacy of specific treatment regimes (Henry & Hill, 1995), but in order to do this adequate outcome measures need to be defined.

In vestibular medicine, patients present with acute illness (for example, viral labyrinthitis, labyrinthine concussion), chronic illness due to a single vestibular insult (for example, poorly compensated peripheral vestibular pathology secondary to ototoxicity, infection, trauma, ischaemia) and acute-on-chronic illness, where the long-term problem is exacerbated by recurrences (for example, benign paroxysmal positional vertigo (BPPV), endolymphatic hydrops, migraine-associated vertigo) (Chapter 5). Rehabilitation is required for those with chronic and acute-on-chronic illness.

## The problems

As vestibular rehabilitation is directed towards the management of vertigo and the improvement of balance, the first thought is that it would be easy to define outcome measures, such as the *severity of the vertigo*, the *frequency of the attacks*, the *severity of the imbalance* and the *number of falls*. However, these outcome measures give no information on disability and little on quality of life. In the rehabilitation of vestibular illness, the major problem is establishing which outcome measures reflect the degree of the patient's improvement or deterioration and also encompass, in a meaningful way, the duration of the improvement in acute-on-chronic illness.

Changes in each of the three parameters of impairment, disability and handicap (WHO, 1980) are important. Changes in impairment are an index of treatment specific to vestibular pathology, but it is now accepted that the patient's own perception should be given the greater consideration. This is in accordance with the guidelines for good clinical practice (WHO, 1988), which stress the importance of assessing therapy on the basis of improvements in the quality of activities in the patient's daily life. It is also well established that measures of vestibular function, as obtained by assessment of the vestibulo-ocular and vestibulo-spinal reflexes, do not correlate with the severity of patients' symptoms (Blakley et al., 1989; Stephens, Hogan & Meredith, 1991; Savundra et al., 1993; Brookes et al., 1994). To a degree, this lack of correlation is a result of the psychological distress which can accompany vertigo (Eagger et al., 1992; Yardley & Putman, 1992), however the perception of vertigo is dependent not only on vestibular function, but also on the integration of vestibular inputs with visual, proprioceptive and tactile inputs, the level of arousal, the cognitive and emotional state of the subject and the degree of dysautonomia (Nakagawa et al., 1993).

Therefore, outcome measures based on the patient's sense of well-being may be influenced as much or more by psychological or social factors as by changes in the level of disability due to the vestibular pathology. For the same reasons the interpretation of responses on the *severity* of vertigo and imbalance is complicated.

A second problem is that careful and successful rehabilitation may lead to a gradual but significant improvement in quality of life, which can be reversed in a moment by a structural change in pathology, for example, due to the movement of debris in BPPV, a further attack of endolymphatic hydrops, or the exposure to a loud sound of a patient with Tullio's phenomenon. Therefore the interpretation of responses based on the *duration* of symptom reduction is complicated not only by the response to rehabilitation but also by the response to the treatment of the underlying pathology.

The interpretation of the *frequency* of attacks following therapy is complicated by avoidance. For example, in BPPV, vertigo is typically induced by particular head movements. Some patients consciously or unconsciously avoid these movements and therefore may report an improvement in quality of life purely as a result of avoidance rather than due to recovery. Equally, patients with imbalance may avoid venturing outdoors or sit in a chair for much of the day, thus avoiding falls, and the outcome measure of the number of falls will give a misleading view of progress due to rehabilitation.

## Potential outcome measures

A number of centres have studied different vestibular parameters in an attempt to assess vestibular compensation. The Hallpike manoeuvre, electronystagmography, caloric and rotation testing, posturography and symptom-rating scales have been used, the last being the one most likely to address the symptomatic status of the patient.

### The Hallpike manoeuvre

This is the definitive test for BPPV, where the characteristic signs have been postulated to be the result of the displacement of otoconia and debris on to the cupula (Schuknecht & Ruby, 1973) or into the long arm (Hall, Ruby & McClure, 1979) of the posterior semicircular canal. However, at any particular time the signs can be normal in patients who still have the condition and the severity of the induced vertigo is not reflected in the induced nystagmus (Savundra et al., 1993). Therefore, a normal response in this test does not necessarily mean the patient has recovered.

## Posturography

Posturography, the measurement of body sway, has been advanced as a possible outcome measure. There are several commercial posturography systems from the relatively inexpensive to the most sophisticated and many laboratories have developed their own customised systems. The parameters of body sway velocity, amplitude and frequency can be measured with the subject either on a static platform with static visual surround or on a moving floor and visual surround, the so-called dynamic posturography, which then allows visual or proprioceptive sway referencing (Figure 12.1) to enhance the differentiation of vestibular, proprioceptive and visual inputs (Norré, 1993) (Figure 12.2).

| Condition | | Vision | Support | Patient Instructions |
|---|---|---|---|---|
| [1] | 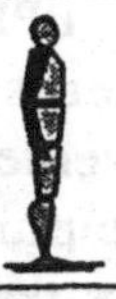 | Normal | Fixed | Stand quietly with your eyes OPEN |
| [2] | 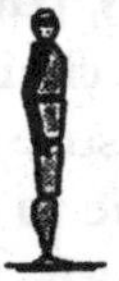 | Absent | Fixed | Stand quietly with your eyes CLOSED |
| [3] | 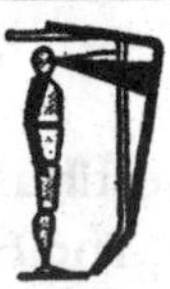 | SwayRef | Fixed | Stand quietly with your eyes OPEN |
| [4] | 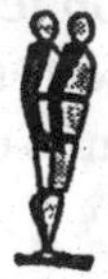 | Normal | SwayRef | Stand quietly with your eyes OPEN |
| [5] | 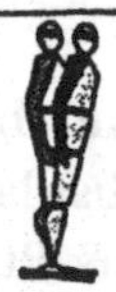 | Absent | SwayRef | Stand quietly with your eyes CLOSED |
| [6] | 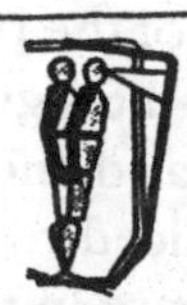 | SwayRef | SwayRef | Stand quietly with your eyes OPEN |

**Figure 12.1** Posturographic test battery. (Reproduced with kind permission: Neurocom. International Inc.)

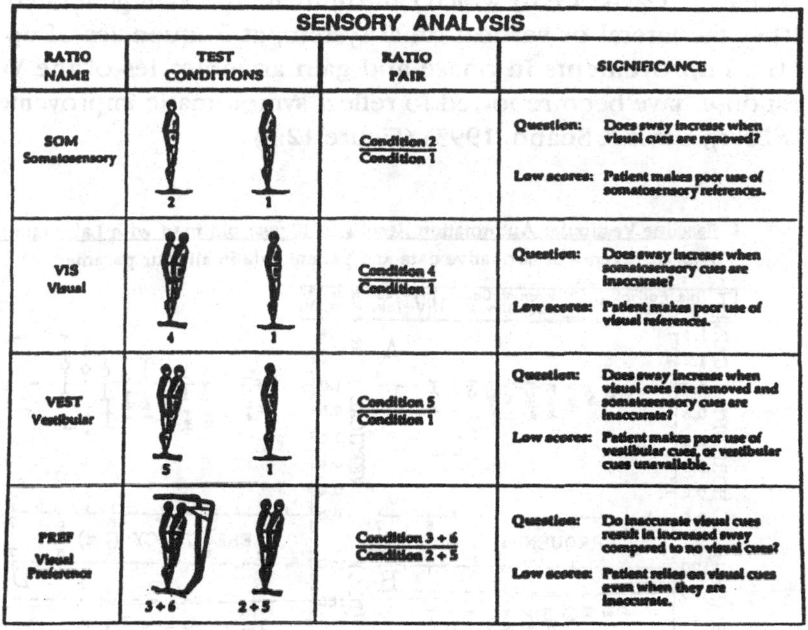

| SENSORY ANALYSIS | | | |
|---|---|---|---|
| RATIO NAME | TEST CONDITIONS | RATIO PAIR | SIGNIFICANCE |
| SOM Somatosensory | 2    1 | Condition 2 / Condition 1 | **Question:** Does sway increase when visual cues are removed? <br><br> **Low scores:** Patient makes poor use of somatosensory references. |
| VIS Visual | 4    1 | Condition 4 / Condition 1 | **Question:** Does sway increase when somatosensory cues are inaccurate? <br><br> **Low scores:** Patient makes poor use of visual references. |
| VEST Vestibular | 5    1 | Condition 5 / Condition 1 | **Question:** Does sway increase when visual cues are removed and somatosensory cues are inaccurate? <br><br> **Low scores:** Patient makes poor use of vestibular cues, or vestibular cues unavailable. |
| PREF Visual Preference | 3 + 6    2 + 5 | Condition 3 + 6 / Condition 2 + 5 | **Question:** Do inaccurate visual cues result in increased sway compared to no visual cues? <br><br> **Low scores:** Patient relies on visual cues even when they are inaccurate. |

**Figure 12.2** Sensory analysis. (Reproduced with kind permission: Equitest Information Pack, Neurocom. International Inc.)

Posturography has been a useful outcome measure in several published studies (Black et al., 1989; Cass, Kartush & Graham, 1991; Shepard et al., 1993), but symptoms do not always correlate with the results (Blakley et al., 1989).

## Measurements of changes in the vestibulo-ocular reflex

Rotational and caloric responses, although of immense diagnostic value in determining the site of lesions, do not correlate with patients' symptoms. The caloric test does not simulate any natural stimulus and the rotation tests do not simulate the environment in which the vestibulo-ocular reflex (VOR) acts in daily life. This is because the VOR naturally acts to stabilise the fovea during walking and running at fundamental frequencies of 2–4 Hz with harmonics extending considerably higher (Grossman et al., 1988), whereas the rotational stimuli routinely used clinically are an order of magnitude less, the limitation being the practicability of building a suitable Barany chair. Moreover, both the caloric and rotational tests assess only lateral canal function and would not be expected to show abnormalities in a symptomatic patient with vertical canal pathology.

An alternative to the Barany chair is active head oscillations (O'Leary & Davis, 1990) which can stimulate the VOR generated by either the lateral or vertical canal system, at frequencies of up to 6 Hz. Improvements in phase and gain asymmetries of the VOR response have been reported to reflect symptomatic improvement (O'Leary, Davis & Suann, 1995) (Figure 12.3).

I. Baseline Vestibular Autorotation Results in 40 year old man with Labyrinthitis.
(N.B. divergence of normative data and patient data in all four parameters.)

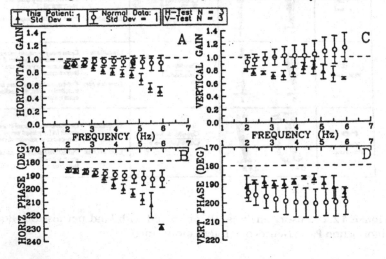

II. Test results after vestibular rehabilitation.
(N.B. Convergence of normative data and test results, together with symptomatic improvement)

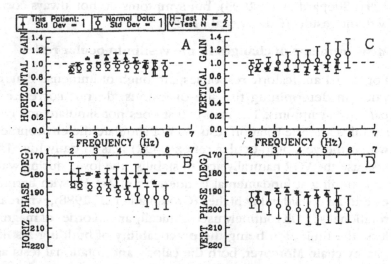

**Figure 12.3** Serial vestibular autorotation results before and after rehabilitation. (Reproduced with kind permission of Dr L Davis O'Leary.)

## Spatial orientation

The ability of subjects to evaluate their rotational orientation by attempting to reorientate a motorised chair following rotational displacements (Metcalfe & Gresty, 1991) has been shown to correlate with questionnaire assessment of vertigo and imbalance (Brookes et al., 1994) and may represent a valuable outcome measure.

## Symptom rating scales

There are discrepancies between the complaints of dizzy patients and objective estimations of balance system function (Hallam & Stephens, 1985) and it is likely therefore that symptom rating scales may be closer to the patient's sense of wellbeing than any laboratory rating scale. There are several symptom scales of value in vestibular rehabilitation (Arenberg & Stahle, 1980; Shepard, Telian & Smith-Wheelock, 1990). The 'vertigo score card' (Savundra et al., 1993) (Figure 12.4) and the 'dizziness handicap inventory' (Jacobson & Newman, 1990) (Figure 12.5) have a high proportion of items concerning the physical causes and triggers for vertigo, whereas the Yardley scales (Yardley et al., 1992) assess the fears and anxieties about the vertigo itself and its implications.

| POSITION CHANGING STIMULI | | |
|---|---|---|
| DO YOU GET DIZZY: | NO | YES |
| 1. BENDING DOWN TO PICK UP SOMETHING FROM THE FLOOR? | | |
| 2. LOOKING UP? | | |
| 3. ON FIRST LAYING IN BED? | | |
| 4. UPON TURNING TO THE LEFT OR RIGHT? | | |
| 5. WHEN WALKING IN THE DARK? | | |
| SUBTOTAL | | |

| VISUAL STIMULI | | |
|---|---|---|
| DO YOU GET DIZZY: | NO | YES |
| 1. WALKING BETWEEN SHELVES IN A SHOP? | | |
| 2. SITTING IN A MOVING VEHICLE? | | |
| 3. WALKING UP OR DOWN STAIRS? | | |
| 4. IRONING STRIPED MATERIAL? | | |
| 5. WALKING UP AN ESCALATOR? | | |
| SUBTOTAL | | |

| TOTAL | |
|---|---|
| | |

No = 1
Yes = 0

Figure 12.4 The vertigo score card.

Yardley's vertigo 'symptom scale' (Figure 12.6) has subscales for acute vertigo, defined as dizziness lasting for at least one hour and accompanied by nausea, ataxia or vomiting; vertigo and imbalance of short duration; autonomic symptoms such as palpitations, breathlessness, faintness, hot or cold spells; and a predisposition to somatisation, whereas the Yardley Handicap Questionnaire (Figure 12.7) describes ways in which vertigo can affect people's lives.

**The Dizziness Handicap Inventory**

1.    Does looking up increase your problem?

2.    Because of your problem, do you feel frustrated?

3.    Because of your problem, do you restrict your travel for business or recreation?

4.    Does walking down the aisle of a supermarket increase your problem?

5.    Because of your problem, do you have difficulty getting into or out of bed?

6.    Does your problem significantly restrict your participation in social activities such as going out to dinner, going to movies, dancing or to parties?

7.    Because of your problem, do you have difficulty reading?

8.    Does performing more ambitious activities like sports, dancing, household chores such as sweeping or putting dishes away increase your problem?

9    Because of your problem, are you afraid to leave your home without having someone to accompany you?

10.    Because of your problem, have you been embarrassed in front of others?

11.    Do quick movements of your head increase your problem?

12.    Because of your problem, do you avoid heights?

13.    Does turning over in bed increase your problem?

14.    Because of your problem, is it difficult for you to do strenuous housework or yardwork?

15.    Because of your problem, are you afraid people may think you are intoxicated?

16.    Because of your problem, is it difficult for you to go for a walk by yourself?

17.    Does walking down a sidewalk increase your problem?

18.    Because of your problem, is it difficult for you to concentrate ?

19.    Because of your problem, is it difficult for you to walk around your house in the dark?

20.    Because of your problem, are you afraid to stay home alone?

21.    Because of your problem, do you feel handicapped?

22.    Has your problem placed stress on your relationships with members of your family or friends?

23.    Because of your problem, are you depressed?

24.    Does your problem interfere with your job or household responsibilities?

25.    Does bending over increase your problem?

**Figure 12.5** The dizziness handicap inventory (Jacobson & Newman, 1990). (Reproduced with kind permission.)

Vertigo Symptom Scale

Please circle the appropriate number to indicate about how many times you have experienced each of the symptoms listed below during the past 12 months (or since the vertigo started, if you have had vertigo for less than one year).
The range of responses:

| 0 | 1 | 2 | 3 | 4 |
|---|---|---|---|---|
| Never | A few times (1-3 times a year) | Several times (4-12 times a year) | Quite often (on average, more than once a month) | Very often (on average, more than once a week) |

How often in the past 12 months have you had the following symptoms:

1. A feeling that things are spinning or moving around, lasting: (PLEASE ANSWER ALL THE CATEGORIES)

|  |  |  |  |  |  |  |
|---|---|---|---|---|---|---|
| a) | - less than 2 minutes | 0 | 1 | 2 | 3 | 4 |
| b) | - up to 20 minutes | 0 | 1 | 2 | 3 | 4 |
| c) | - 20 minutes to 1 hour | 0 | 1 | 2 | 3 | 4 |
| d) | - several hours | 0 | 1 | 2 | 3 | 4 |
| e) | - more than 12 hours | 0 | 1 | 2 | 3 | 4 |

2. Pains in the heart or chest region — 0 1 2 3 4
3. Hot and cold spells — 0 1 2 3 4
4. Unsteadiness so severe that you actually fall — 0 1 2 3 4
5. Nausea (feeling sick), stomach churning — 0 1 2 3 4
6. Tension/soreness in your muscles — 0 1 2 3 4
7. A feeling of being light headed, "swimmy" or giddy, — 0 1 2 3 4
   lasting: (PLEASE ANSWER ALL THE CATEGORIES)

|  |  |  |  |  |  |  |
|---|---|---|---|---|---|---|
| a) | - less than 2 minutes | 0 | 1 | 2 | 3 | 4 |
| b) | - up to 20 minutes | 0 | 1 | 2 | 3 | 4 |
| c) | - 20 minutes to 1 hour | 0 | 1 | 2 | 3 | 4 |
| d) | - several hours | 0 | 1 | 2 | 3 | 4 |
| e) | - more than 12 hours | 0 | 1 | 2 | 3 | 4 |

8. Trembling shivering — 0 1 2 3 4
9. Feeling of pressure in the ear(s) — 0 1 2 3 4
10. Heart pounding or fluttering — 0 1 2 3 4
11. Vomiting — 0 1 2 3 4
12. Heavy feeling in arms or legs — 0 1 2 3 4
13. Visual disturbances (e.g. blurring spots before the eyes) — 0 1 2 3 4
14. Headaches or feeling of pressure in the head — 0 1 2 3 4
15. Unable to stand or walk properly without support — 0 1 2 3 4
16. Difficulty breathing, short of breath — 0 1 2 3 4
17. Loss of concentration or memory — 0 1 2 3 4
18. Feeling unsteady, about to lose balance, lasting: (PLEASE ANSWER ALL THE CATEGORIES)

|  |  |  |  |  |  |  |
|---|---|---|---|---|---|---|
| a) | - less than 2 minutes | 0 | 1 | 2 | 3 | 4 |
| b) | - up to 20 minutes | 0 | 1 | 2 | 3 | 4 |
| c) | - 20 minutes to 1 hour | 0 | 1 | 2 | 3 | 4 |
| d) | - several hours | 0 | 1 | 2 | 3 | 4 |
| e) | - more than 12 hours | 0 | 1 | 2 | 3 | 4 |

19. Tingling, prickling or numbness in parts of the body — 0 1 2 3 4
20. Pains in the lower part of your back — 0 1 2 3 4
21. Excessive sweating — 0 1 2 3 4
22. Feeling faint, about to black out — 0 1 2 3 4

**Figure 12.6** The Vertigo 'symptom scale' (Yardley et al., 1992). (Reproduced with kind permission.)

## Vertigo Handicap Questionnaire

The statements below describe ways in which vertigo can affect people's lives. Throughout the questionnaire the word "vertigo" is used to describe the feelings which you may call dizziness, giddiness or unsteadiness. We would like you to indicate whether vertigo has affected your life in any of these ways by circling a number between 0 and 4. The response categories are:

| 0 | 1 | 2 | 3 | 4 |
|---|---|---|---|---|
| always | often | sometimes | occasionally | never |

*Scoring and administration.* To obtain the total handicap score (out of 80) simply sum responses to items 1 to 25 of the VHQ, *after first reversing the scores on the asterisked items* (so that 0=4, 4=0, etc).

*Statistical properties and normative values* (based on a sample of 120 outpatients referred for investigation of balance disorder). The VHQ has very good reliability (alpha = .86); the mean handicap score was 46.3 with a standard deviation of 17.24. Test-retest reliability of the VHQ has been shown to be good.

Please read each statement and then circle a number to indicate how much of the time (if at all) vertigo affects your life in the way at present.

1.  I find that the vertigo does affect my life.       (Never) 0 1 2 3 4 5 (Always)
2.  I can still take part in active leisure             (Never) 0 1 2 3 4 5 (Always)
    pursuits (e.g. swimming, dancing, sports).
3.  Some of my friends or relations get                (Never) 0 1 2 3 4 5 (Always)
    impatient because of the vertigo.
4.  I can move around quickly and freely               (Never) 0 1 2 3 4 5 (Always)
5.  I feel less confident than used to.                (Never) 0 1 2 3 4 5 (Always)
6.  I am happy to go out alone.                        (Never) 0 1 2 3 4 5 (Always)
7.  My vertigo means that my family life is            (Never) 0 1 2 3 4 5 (Always)
    restricted.
8.  I find some of my less active hobbies              (Never) 0 1 2 3 4 5 (Always)
    difficult. (e.g. sewing, reading)
9.  I am still able to travel despite the vertigo.     (Never) 0 1 2 3 4 5 (Always)
10. I try to avoid bending over.                       (Never) 0 1 2 3 4 5 (Always)
11. My family takes the vertigo in its stride.         (Never) 0 1 2 3 4 5 (Always)
12. My friends are unsure how to react and do          (Never) 0 1 2 3 4 5 (Always)
    not really understand.
13. I think there may be something seriously           (Never) 0 1 2 3 4 5 (Always)
    wrong with me.
14.* People are understanding about the                (Never) 0 1 2 3 4 5 (Always)
    problems that the vertigo causes.
15. I get anxious in case I have an unexpected         (Never) 0 1 2 3 4 5 (Always)
    attack of vertigo.
16.* During an attack of vertigo I can carry on        (Never) 0 1 2 3 4 5 (Always)
    with whatever I am doing.
17. I find the attacks frightening.                    (Never) 0 1 2 3 4 5 (Always)
18.* I am able to walk long distances.                 (Never) 0 1 2 3 4 5 (Always)
19. The vertigo worries me.                            (Never) 0 1 2 3 4 5 (Always)
20. I avoid making plans in advance in case I          (Never) 0 1 2 3 4 5 (Always)
    cannot get there on the day.
21.* I find I can carry out every day activities       (Never) 0 1 2 3 4 5 (Always)
    without difficulty (e.g. shopping, gardening,
    jobs around the house).
22. I am afraid of spoiling things for others.         (Never) 0 1 2 3 4 5 (Always)
23. I get rather depressed because of the vertigo.     (Never) 0 1 2 3 4 5 (Always)
24. During an attack of vertigo, if I sit down I       (Never) 0 1 2 3 4 5 (Always)
    am fine.
25. During an attack of vertigo, in public I get       (Never) 0 1 2 3 4 S (Always)
    embarrassed.
26. Are you currently employed? (Please Tick)                          Yes No

If you answered "Yes" to question 26 please answer question b) and c) only.
If you answered "No" to question 26 please answer question a) only.

a) Did you give up work because of vertigo?                            Yes No
b) Have you changed the type of work you do because of vertigo?        Yes No
c) Does vertigo cause you any difficulties at work?                    Yes No

**Figure 12.7** The Vertigo Handicap Questionnaire (Yardley et al., 1992). (Reproduced with kind permission.)

# Summary

It is of great importance to establish the comparative value of vestibular rehabilitation regimes. The difficulty is determining outcome measures which are sensitive to changes in vestibular function and which also reflect the patient's sense of wellbeing. The Hallpike manoeuvre in BPPV and the vestibular autorotation test, dynamic posturography and the psychophysical test of the subjective awareness of rotation are likely to be useful clinical outcome measures, whereas validated symptom rating scales will measure changes in disability, handicap and quality of life. It is important to include a combination of these outcome measures to provide a satisfactory index of the value of an intervention regime.

# Chapter 13
# Setting up a service

ROSALYN A DAVIES

## Introduction

It is well recognised that dizziness is a prevalent symptom, with Roydhouse (1974) reporting that 30% of the population has had a medical consultation for this symptom by the age of 65 years, and Yardley and Luxon (1994) reporting that five per 1000 population consult their GP each year for true vertigo, and 10 per 1000 for dizziness. It is also established that a minor vestibular impairment can confer major disability and handicap if left unmanaged (Yardley, 1994; Jacobson & Newman, 1990; Shepard et al., 1993). Other sequelae include psychiatric morbidity, such as depression and panic disorder, loss of time from work and ultimately early retirement on the grounds of ill health (Eagger et al., 1992).

There are clear financial implications arising from poor management of recurrent dizziness. These can be considered in terms of the cost to the individual, the cost to the National Health Service (NHS) as well as in the cost to the state. The individual's own morbidity will not only affect his quality of life, but also affect his capacity to earn a living. The costs to the NHS involve multiple visits to the GP, but in addition multiple referrals to hospital specialists where there may be no provision for vestibular rehabilitation, i.e. general physicians, neurologists and some ENT surgeons. The cost to the state is in providing Disability Allowance when patients' symptoms affect their activities of daily living rendering them disabled or handicapped.

## Multidisciplinary approach

The World Health Organization schema (WHO, 1980) for disablement describes the pathway whereby an aetiological factor leading to pathology results in impairment and may go on to produce disability and handicap (Chapter 2). This pathway can be equally well applied to vestibular dysfunction as to any other impairment. The appropriate response to providing a service to counteract the development of disability and handicap needs to be multidisciplinary.

To recognise the underlying vestibular pathology and identify an aetiological agent requires formal medical assessment in the first instance with instigation of any medical/surgical treatment as appropriate. Further evaluation becomes investigation-orientated requiring appropriately trained professionals able to carry out a full audio–vestibular test battery. The next stage, rehabilitation, may require any of a variety of therapeutic approaches (Shumway-Cook & Horak, 1990). Physical exercises, such as the Cawthorne Cooksey exercises, may be required to promote central compensation. Particle-repositioning manoeuvres, such as the Epley procedure, may be required to clear otoconial debris from the posterior semicircular canal in patients with benign paroxysmal positional vertigo (BPPV) (Chapter 9). Breathing and/or relaxation exercises may be required for patients who hyperventilate either as a primary factor in the generation of dizziness, or secondarily as an anxiety response to induced dizziness (Chapters 6 and 8). Behaviour therapy may be required for those patients who demonstrate avoidance behaviour, avoiding the situations which provoke their symptoms of dizziness or imbalance (Chapter 7). Where there is an excessive focus on the balance symptoms, cognitive therapy may be appropriate. All these approaches are covered by the term 'vestibular rehabilitation'.

## Vestibular rehabilitation and key personnel

For each of the stages in the provision of a vestibular rehabilitation service, different professionals are required (Beynon & Baguley, 1995) (Table 13.1).

Table 13.1 Multidisciplinary approach

| | |
|---|---|
| Diagnosis: | |
| general medical | audiological physician/ENTsurgeon/ |
| otological | neurologist |
| neurological | |
| | |
| Assessment/investigation: | |
| audiological test battery | audiological scientist/audiological |
| vestibular test battery | technician/trained nurse |
| dizziness simulation tests | |
| | |
| Rehabilitation: | |
| Cawthorne Cooksey exercises | physiotherapist/audiological scientist/ |
| particle-repositioning manoeuvres | audiological technician/hearing therapist |
| breathing exercises | |
| relaxation exercises | |
| behavioural/cognitive | psychologist/psychiatric nurse |
| psychotherapy | |

Patients with recurrent dizziness present not only with primary symptoms of vertigo, imbalance and blurred vision but also with secondary symptoms of neck pain, muscle tension, fatigue and low mood (Shumway-Cook & Horak, 1990). The formal evaluation of these symptoms requires a comprehensive history, including reference to general medical symptoms and psychological symptoms, as well as otological and neurological symptoms. The physical examination, including otoscopy, tuning fork tests, eye movement examination, positional testing, gait assessment, as well as a visual assessment and neurological/musculo-skeletal assessment, is necessary. The diagnosis and investigation of aetiological agents is the role of medically trained personnel and traditionally this is an ENT surgeon or an audiological physician. Further assessment and evaluation by audio–vestibular testing is traditionally carried out by the audiological scientist/technician. The importance of assessing any accompanying audiological dysfunction, as well as characterising any vestibular impairment will then determine the next stages of vestibular rehabilitation. Therapeutic options include physical exercise regimes, breathing exercises, relaxation exercises, as well as behaviour or cognitive therapy. The physiotherapist generally instructs the dizzy patient in Cawthorne Cooksey exercises, or Brandt–Darroff exercises. The Epley manoeuvre for particle-repositioning in BPPV is best carried out by a medically trained person in view of rare, but unpleasant complications (Chapter 9). Relaxation and breathing exercises may be taught by physiotherapists, a nurse appropriately trained in this area, or appropriately trained hearing therapists. The area of behaviour and cognitive therapy falls into the realm of the nurse, behaviour therapist or psychologist. Thus, a team approach with good communication between all involved becomes the ideal framework for establishing a successful vestibular rehabilitation service.

## Audio–vestibular test equipment

A comprehensive test battery to investigate the dizzy patient requires access to both audiological and vestibular tests (Table 13.2).

Table 13.2 Balance centre testing

Pure tone audiometry (PTA)
Admittance testing
Acoustic brainstem response (ABR)
Electronystagmography (ENG) chart recorder
Visual/vestibular stimuli (rotary chair)
Caloric testing
Posturography with sensory organisation testing

Pure tone audiometry (PTA) and admittance testing provide screening for peripheral auditory function and, where an abnormality is detected, further evaluation with auditory-evoked brainstem responses (ABR) may be required. From the vestibular point of view an electronystagmography (ENG) chart recorder to document the eye movements in response to gaze testing, smooth pursuit and caloric stimuli is required. Where funding is available, a rotary chair with computer-driven and analysed visual/vestibular stimuli allows documentation and quantification of nystagmus, smooth pursuit, saccades, optokinetic nystagmus (OKN) and vestibulo-ocular reflex (VOR) suppression, all helpful in differentiating otological from neurological dizziness. Ideally, posturography should be available, including a programme of sensory organisation testing. Again, where funding is available, the Equitest is probably the most sophisticated way to assess balance under different sensory test conditions and this equipment can also document the latency of motor responses to translational stimuli, i.e. allowing some evaluation of the integrity of effector pathways. Other forceplate posturography platforms can be combined with facilities to modulate visual and proprioceptive information to provide a test of sensory organisation. Objective information on patient sway and sensory organisation allows for monitoring responses to rehabilitation interventions. Of all the test equipment available, posturography is probably the most suitable tool with which to guide rehabilitation strategies and monitor serial changes in balance function, although the more recent advances in VOR assessment by use of vestibular autorotation testing (Chapter 12) also shows promise.

## Selling the service

The level of funding available to set up a rehabilitation service is often related to purchaser interest in the service and the importance of selling the success of a rehabilitation service becomes fundamental. Outcome measures are the standard way of determining success of a medical intervention. *The Health of the Nation* strategy document (HMSO, 1992) focuses on rehabilitation and returning patients to work, and research in this area of effectiveness of rehabilitation strategies is presently given financial backing.

Outcome measures include both subjective assessments as well as objective testing. Vertigo and disability questionnaires, such as the vertigo symptom scale (Yardley, 1994)) and the dizziness handicap inventory (Jacobson & Newman, 1990) provide useful tools to evaluate dizziness both before, as a baseline measure, and after rehabilitation. These are disease-specific questionnaires and are best used in conjunction with a generic questionnaire, such as is used commonly in public health medicine, for example, the Short Form 36, to evaluate general health effects. These measures allow the impact of the symptom on the performance and lifestyle of the individual to be measured in a validated way. As mentioned above, objective assessment of rehabilitation success includes posturography (sensory organisation testing). This particular tool has the advantage of identifying false balance strategies requiring retraining and helping to convey different approaches to improve outcome, that is some patients are evaluated as being visually dependent, suggesting an over-reliance on the visual system to substitute for impaired vestibular input. Vestibular signs (Stephens, Hogan & Meredith, 1991) and standard vestibular tests using caloric irrigations and rotary chair tests have not been shown to be of great value when compared with subjective assessments of improvement in dizziness status (Yardley, 1994).

## Referral protocols

To maximise the efficiency of a vestibular rehabilitation service, the purchaser needs clear referral protocols to identify candidates suitable for a rehabilitation programme (British Association of Audiological Physicians, 1994). The protocols recommended are identified in Table 13.3.

Table 13.3 Referral protocols

| |
| --- |
| Vertigo/dizziness of >6 weeks' duration |
| Vertigo and hearing loss/tinnitus |
| Vertigo and neurological symptoms |

For each of these three categories, different primary assessment and investigation protocols are recommended, respectively:

- Vertigo/dizziness of more than six weeks' duration: PTA and admittance studies with ENG and calorics.
- Vertigo and hearing loss/tinnitus: PTA, admittance testing (±) ABRs, ENG and calorics and possibly magnetic resonance imaging (MRI).
- Vertigo and neurological symptoms: PTA, admittance testing and ABRs, ENG, calorics. Clearly, additional investigation may be required with imaging in the form of computer tomography (CT) scanning or MRI or with EEG or cardiological assessment with ECG, 24-hour ECG or Echo.

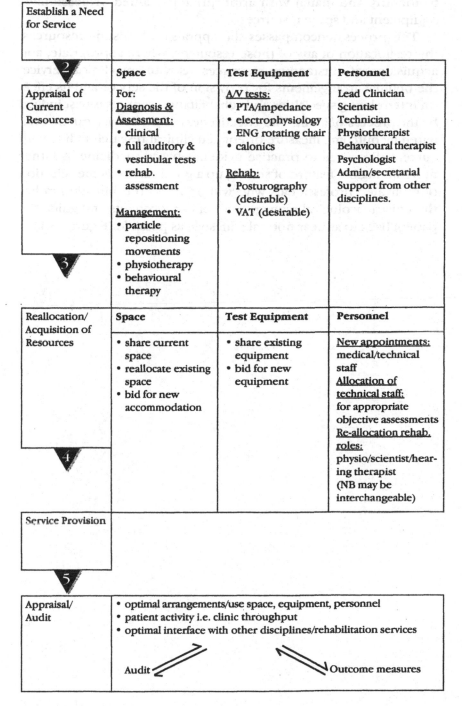

**Figure 13.1** Setting up a vestibular rehabilitation service.

The professional faced with setting up a service has many tasks to identify and match with appropriately trained professionals, equipment and space resources.

This process encompasses the appraisal of existing resources, the reallocation of any of those resources, where appropriate, and acquisition of outstanding resources. As with any clinical service, the optimal arrangements for provision of the service and its effect on interrelating specialties and rehabilitation services is best judged by the process of audit. The effectiveness of the service can be evaluated by outcome measure-orientated clinical research in line with current directives to practise evidence-based medicine. A rather more intangible feature of setting up a good service is the selection of motivated professionals who will prioritise rehabilitation rather than pharmacological management of dizzy patients and guide the patient back to as near normal a lifestyle as possible (Figure 13.1).

# References

Anderson JH, Soechting JF, Terzuolo CA (1979) Role of vestibular inputs in the organisation of motor output to the forelimb extensors. Progress in Brain Research 50, 582–596.

Arenberg IK, Stahle J (1980) Staging Ménière's disease (or any inner ear dysfunction) and the use of the vertigogram. Otolaryngologic Clinics of North America 13, 643–656.

Axelsson A (1974) The blood supply of the inner ear in mammals. In WC Kiedel, WD Neff (eds) Handbook of Sensory Physiology. Auditory System Volume V Part I. Berlin: Springer-Verlag, pp. 213–260.

Baloh TW (1996) Benign positional vertigo. In: RW Baloh, M Halmagyi (eds). Handbook of Neuro-otology/Vestibular System. New York: Oxford University Press. pp. 328–339.

Baloh RW, Honrubia V (1990) Clinical Neurophysiology of the Vestibular System. Philadelphia, PN: Davis FA.

Baloh RW, Jacobson K, Honrubia V (1993) Horizontal semicircular canal variant of benign positional vertigo. Neurology 43, 2542–2549.

Barber HJ, Leigh JR (1988) Benign and not so benign positional vertigo; diagnosis and treatment. Cited in JA Freeman, JA Nairne (1995) Using a class setting to teach Cawthorne Cooksey exercises as a means of vestibular rehabilitation. Physiotherapy 81, 374–379.

Bass C (1990) Physical Symptoms and Psychological Illness. Oxford: Blackwell Scientific.

Békésy G (1966) Pressure and shearing forces as stimuli of labyrinthine epithelium. Archives of Otolaryngology 84, 122–130.

Bender MB (1965) Oscillopsia. Archives of Neurology 13, 204–213.

Benson H (1975) The relaxation response. Cited in Health Media & Education Centre (1987) Teaching people to unwind: relaxation and stress management techniques. Department of New South Wales: State Health Publication No. (HMEC) 87-022, p. 8.

Beynon GJ, Baguley DM (1995) The case of setting up a vestibular rehabilitation service. Balance Interest Group Document 3. British Society of Audiology.

Black FO, Schupert CL, Horak FB, Nashner LM (1988) Abnormal postural control associated with peripheral vestibular disorders. In: O Pompeiano, JHJ Allum (eds). Progress in Brain Research. London: Elsevier Science, pp. 263–275.

Black FO, Schupert CL, Peterka RJ, Nashner LM (1989). Effects of unilateral loss of vestibular function on the vestibulo-ocular reflex and postural control. Annals of Otology, Rhinology and Laryngology 98, 884–889.

Blakley BW, Barber HO, Tomlinson RD, Stoyanoft S, Mai MI (1989) On the search for markers of poor vestibular compensation. Otolaryngology, Head and Neck Surgery 101, 572–577.

Bles W, De Jon JMB, Rasmussens JJ (1984) Postural and oculomotor signs in labyrinthine defective subjects. Acta Otolaryngologica (Suppl.) 406, 101–104.

Bonner D, Ron M, Chalder T, Butler S, Wessley S (1994) Chronic fatigue syndrome: a follow-up study. Journal of Neurology, Neurosurgery and Psychiatry 57, 617–621.

Borello-France DF, Whitney SL, Herdman SJ (1994) Assessment of vestibular hypofunction. In: SJ Herdman (ed.). Vestibular Rehabilitation. Philadelphia: FA Davis, pp. 247–279.

Bottini G, Sterzi R, Paulesu E, Vallar G, Cappa SF, Ermino F, Passingham RE, Frith CD, Frackowiack RSJ (1994) Identification of the central vestibular projections in man: a positron emission tomography activation study. Experimental Brain Research 99, 164–169.

Brandt T (1990) Downbeat nystagmus/vertigo syndrome. In: Vertigo: Its Multisensory Syndromes. London: Springer-Verlag, pp. 99–107.

Brandt T, Daroff RB (1980) Physical therapy for benign paroxysmal positional vertigo. Archives of Otolaryngology 106, 484–485.

Brandt T, Dieterich M (1993) Vestibular falls. Journal of Vestibular Research 3, 3–14.

Brandt T, Steddin S (1993). Current view of the mechanism of benign paroxysmal positional vertigo: cupulolithiasis or canalithiasis? Journal of Vestibular Research 3, 373–382.

Brandt T, Buchele W, Arnold F (1977) Arthrokinetic nystagmus and ego-motion sensation. Experimental Brain Research 30, 331–338.

Brandt T, Huppert D, Dieterich M (1994) Phobic postural vertigo: a first follow-up. Journal of Neurology 241, 191–195.

British Association of Audiological Physicians (1994) Guidelines for the Care of Patients with Hearing Loss, Tinnitus and Imbalance in the United Kingdom. Cardiff: BAAP.

Bronstein AM (1995) Visual vertigo syndrome: clinical and posturography findings. Journal of Neurology, Neurosurgery and Psychiatry 59, 472–476.

Bronstein AM, Hood JD (1987) Oscillopsia of peripheral vestibular origin: central and cervical compensatory mechanisms. Acta Otolaryngologica 104, 307–314.

Bronstein AM, Miller DH, Rudge P, Kendall BE (1987) Downbeating nystagmus: magnetic resonance imaging and neuro-otological findings. Journal of Neurological Science 81, 173–184.

Bronstein A, Rinne T, Gresty M, Rudge P, Luxon LM (1996) Bilateral loss of vestibular function. Acta Otolaryngologica (Suppl.) 520, 247–250.

Brookes GB, Faldon M, Kanayama R, Nakamura T, Gresty MA (1994) Recovery from unilateral vestibular nerve section in human subjects evaluated by physiological, psychological and questionnaire assessments. Acta Otolaryngologica Supplementum 513, 40–48.

Brown JJ (1990) A systematic approach to the dizzy patient. Neurologic Clinics 8, 209–224.

Buchelle W, Brandt T, Degner D (1983) Ataxia and oscillopsia in downbeat-nystagmus vertigo syndrome. Advances in Otorhinolaryngology 30, 291–297.

Calza L, Giardino L, Zanni M, Galetti R, Parchi P, Galetti G (1989) Involvement of cholinergic and GABA-ergic systems in vestibular compensation. In Lacour M, Toupet M, Denise P, Christen Y (eds). Vestibular Compensation: Facts, Theories and Clinical Perspectives. Paris: Elsevier, pp. 189–199.

Cannon WB (1953) Bodily Changes in Pain, Hunger, Fear and Rage. Boston, MA: Charles T Branford.

Caplan LR (1986) Vertebrobasilar disease. In: HJM Barnett, JP Mohr, BM Stein, FM Yatsu (eds). Stroke: Pathophysiology, Diagnosis and Management. New York: Churchill Livingstone.

Carnahan H (1992) Eye, head and hand coordination during manual aiming. In: L Proteau, D Elliot (eds). Vision and Motor Control. London: Elsevier Science, pp. 179–196.

Cass SP, Goshgarian HG (1991) Vestibular compensation after labyrinthectomy and vestibular neurectomy in cats. Otolaryngology — Head and Neck Surgery 104, 14–19.

Cass SP, Kartush JM, Graham MD (1991) Clinical assessment of postural stability following vestibular nerve section. Laryngoscope 101, 1056–1059.

Cawthorne TE (1945) Vestibular injuries. Proceedings of the Royal Society of Medicine 39, 270–273.

Christie RV (1935) Some types of respiration in the neuroses. Quarterly Journal of Medicine 16, 427–432.

Clark DB, Hirsch BE, Smith MG, Furman JMR, Jacob RG (1994) Panic in otolaryngology patients presenting with dizziness or hearing loss. American Journal of Psychiatry 151, 1223–1225.

Cochrane AL (1972) Effectiveness and Efficiency: Random Reflections on Health Services. London: Nuffield Provincial Hospitals Trust.

Cohen B, Suzuki JI, Bender MB (1964) Eye movements from semicircular canal nerve stimulation in the cat. Annals of Otology, Rhinology and Laryngology 73, 153–169.

Cooksey FS (1945) Rehabilitation of vestibular injuries. Proceedings of the Royal Society of Medicine 39, 273–278.

Courjon JH, Jeannerod M, Ossuzio I, Schmid R (1977) The role of vision in compensation of vestibulo-ocular reflex after hemilabyrinthectomy in the cat. Experimental Brain Research 28, 235–248.

Curthoys IS, Halmagyi GM (1995) Vestibular compensation: a review of the occulomotor, neural and clinical consequences of unilateral vestibular loss. Journal of Vestibular Research 5, 67–107.

Da Costa JM (1871) On irritable heart: a clinical study of a form of functional cardiac disorder and its consequences. American Journal of Medical Sciences 61, 17–52.

Darlington CL, Smith PF, Hubbard JI (1989) Neuronal activity in the guinea-pig medial vestibular nucleus in vitro following chronic unilateral labyrinthectomy. Neuroscience Letters 105, 143–148.

Davies RA, Savundra PA (1997) Clinical examination of vestibular symptoms Chapter 2. In: Scott Brown's Otolaryngology Volume 2. London: Butterworths, pp. 1–40.

Dichgans J, Nauck B, Wolpert E (1973) The influence of attention, vigilance and stimulus area on optokinetic and vestibular nystagmus and voluntary saccades. In Zikmund V (ed). The Oculomotor System and Brain

Functions. London: Butterworths, pp. 279–294.

Dieringer N, Kunzle H, Precht W (1984) Increased projections of dorsal root fibres to vestibular nuclei after hemilabyrinthectomy in the frog. Experimental Brain Research 55, 574–578.

Dieterich M, Brandt T (1990) Postural imbalance and subjective visual vertical in medullary infarctions. In: T Brandt et al. (eds). Disorders of Posture and Gait. New York: George Thieme Verlag, pp. 419–423.

Di Fabio RP (1995) Sensitivity and specificity of platform posturography for identifying patients with vestibular dysfunction. Physical Therapy 75, 260–305.

Dix MR (1974) Treatment of vertigo. Physiotherapy 60, 380–384.

Dix MR (1976) The physiological basis and practical value of head exercises in the treatment of vertigo. Practitioner 217, 919.

Dix MR (1979) The rationale and technique of head exercises in the treatment of vertigo. Acta Otolaryngologica Belgica 33, 370–384.

Dix MR (1984) Rehabilitation of vertigo. In: MR Dix, JD Hood (eds). Vertigo. New York: Wiley & Sons, pp. 23–39.

Dix MR, Hallpike CS (1952) Pathology, symptomatology and diagnosis of certain common disorders of the vestibular system. Proceedings of the Royal Society of Medicine 45, 341–354.

Dix R, Hallpike CS (1952) The pathology, symptomatology and diagnosis of certain common disorders of the vestibular system. Annals of Otology 61, 987–1016.

Dohlman G (1938) On the mechanism of transmission into nystagmus on stimulation of the semicircular canals. Acta Otolaryngologica 26, 425–442.

Drachman DB, Hart CW (1972) An approach to the dizzy patient. Neurology 22, 323–334.

Eagger S, Luxon LM, Davies RA, Coelho A, Ron MA (1992) Psychiatric morbidity in peripheral vestibular disease; a clinical and neuro-otological study. Journal of Neurology, Neurosurgery and Psychiatry 55, 383–387.

van Egmond AAJ, Groen JJ, Jongkees LBW (1948) The turning test with small regulable stimuli. Journal of Laryngology and Otology 62, 63–69.

Epley JM (1992) The canalith repositioning procedure: for treatment of benign paroxysmal positional vertigo. Otolaryngology, Head and Neck Surgery 107, 399–404.

Errington ML, Lynch MA, Bliss TVP (1987) Long-term potentiation in the dentate nucleus: induction and increased glutamate release are blocked by D(–) aminophosphonovalerate. Neuroscience 20, 279–284.

Evidence-based Medicine Working Group (1992) Evidence-based medicine. A new approach to the teaching of medicine. Journal of the American Medical Association 268, 2420–2425.

Ewald JR (1892) Physiologisch Untersuchungen uber das Endorgan des Nervus Octavus. Wiesbaden: Bergmann.

Fernandez C, Goldberg JM (1971) Physiology of peripheral neurons innervating semicircular canals of squirrel monkey. II. Response to sinusoidal stimulation and dynamics of peripheral vestibular system. Journal of Neurophysiology 34, 661–675.

Fernandez C, Goldberg JM (1976) Physiology of peripheral neurons innervating otolith organs of the squirrel monkey. Journal of Neurophysiology 39, 970–1008.

Fetter M, Zee DS, Proctor LR (1988). Effect of lack of vision and of occipital lobectomy upon recovery from unilateral labyrinthectomy in rhesus monkey. Journal of Neurophysiology 59, 394–407.

Fisher CM (1982) Lacunar strokes and infarcts: a review. Neurology 32, 871.

Fitzgerald G, Hallpike CS (1942) Studies in human vestibular function: 1. Observations on the directional preponderance ("Nystagmusbereitschaft" of caloric nystagmus resulting from cerebral lesions. Brain 65, 115–137.

Flock A, Cheung HC (1977) Actin filaments in sensory hairs of inner ear receptor cells. Journal of Cell Biology 75, 339–343.

Freeman JA, Nairne J (1995) Using a class setting to teach Cawthorne Cooksey exercises as a means of vestibular rehabilitation. Physiotherapy 81, 74–79.

Fuchs AF, Kimm J (1975) Unit activity in vestibular nucleus of the alert monkey during horizontal angular acceleration and eye movement. Journal of Neurophysiology 38, 1140–1161.

Fujino A, Toumasu K, Okamoto M, Naganuma H, Hoshino I, Arai M, Yoneda S (1996) Vestibular training for acute unilateral vestibular disturbances: its efficacy in comparison with antivertigo drug. Acta Otolaryngologica 524, 21–26.

Furman JF (1995) Role of posturography in the management of vestibular patients. Otolaryngology, Head and Neck Surgery 112, 8–15.

Gacek RR (1978) Further observations on posterior ampullary nerve transection for positional vertigo. Annals of Otology, Rhinology and Laryngology 87, 300–305.

Gelder MC, Bancroft JH, Gath D, Jonstone CDW, Mathews AM (1973) Specific and non-specific factors in behavioural therapy. British Journal of Psychiatry 123, 445–462.

Gill-Body KM, Krebs DE (1994) Locomotor stability problems associated with vestibulopathy: assessment and treatment. Physical Therapy Practice 3, 232–245.

Girardi M, Horst P, Konrad MD (1996) Management of benign paroxysmal positional vertigo ORL. Head and Neck Nursing 14, 25–30.

Goldberg D, Gask L, O'Dowd T (1989) Treatment of somatisation: teaching techniques of reattribution. Journal of Psychosomatic Research 33, 689–695.

Goldman A (1922) Clinical tetany by forced expiration. Journal of the American Medical Association 78, 1193–1195.

Gonshor A, Melvill Jones G (1976) Extreme vestibulo-ocular adaptation induced by prolonged optical reversal of vision. Journal of Physiology 256, 381–414.

Green J, Wintfield N, Sharkey P, Passman LJ (1990) The importance of severity of illness in assessing hospital mortality. Journal of the American Medical Association 263, 241–246.

Gresty MA, Trinder E, Leech J (1976) Perception of everyday visual environments during saccadic eye movements. Aviation Space & Environmental Medicine 47, 991–992.

Gresty MA, Barratt H, Rudge P (1986) Analysis of downbeat nystagmus. Otolithic versus semicircular canal influences. Archives of Neurology 43, 52–55.

Grossman GE, Leigh RJ (1990) Instability of gaze during locomotion in patients with deficient vestibular function. Annals of Neurology 27, 528–532.

Grossman GE, Leigh RJ, Abel LA, Lanska DJ, Thurston SE (1988) Frequency and velocity of rotational head movements during locomotion. Experimental

Brain Research 70, 470–476.

Guedry FE (1974) Psychophysics of vestibular sensation. In HH Kornhuber (ed.). Psychophysics, Applied Aspects and General Interpretations. Volume VI Vestibular System (Part 2) Handbook of Sensory Physiology. Berlin: Springer-Verlag, pp. 3–154.

Guitton D (1992) Control of eye–head coordination during orienting gaze shifts. Trends in Neuroscience 15, 174–179.

Haddad GM, Demer JL, Robinson DAS (1980) The effect of lesions of the dorsal cap of the inferior olive on the vestibulo-ocular and optokinetic system of the cat. Brain Research 185, 265–275.

Haldane JS, Poulton EP (1908) The effects of want of oxygen on respiration. Journal of Physiology 37, 390–407.

Hall SF, Ruby RRF, McClure JA (1979) The mechanics of benign paroxysmal vertigo. Journal of Otolaryngology 8, 151–158.

Hallam RS, Stephens SDG (1985) Vestibular disorder and emotional distress. Journal of Psychosomatic Research 29, 407–413.

Harada V (1979) Formation area of statoconia. Scanning Electron Microscope 3, 963–966.

Health Media & Education Centre (1987) Teaching People to Unwind: Relaxation and Stress Management Techniques. Department of New South Wales: State Health Publication No. (HMEC) 87-022.

Hecker HC, Haug CO, Herndon JW (1974) Treatment of the vertiginous patient using Cawthorne's vestibular exercises. Laryngoscope 84, 2065–2072.

Henry D, Hill S (1995) Comparing treatments. British Medical Journal 310, 1279.

Herdman SJ (1994) Assessment and management of bilateral vestibular loss. In: S Herdman (ed.). Vestibular Rehabilitation. Philadelphia: FA Davis, pp. 316–329.

Herdman S (1995) Vestibular adaptation exercises and recovery: acute stage after acoustic neuroma resection. Otolargyngology, Head and Neck Surgery 113, 77–87.

Herdman SJ, Tusa RJ, Zee DS, Proctor LR, Mattox DE (1993) Single treatment approaches to benign positional vertigo. Achives of Otolaryngology and Head and Neck Surgery 119, 450–454.

Herdman S, Borello-France DF, Whitney SL (1994) Treatment of vestibular hypofunction. In: S Herdman (ed.). Vestibular Rehabilitation. Philadelphia: FA Davis, pp. 287–313.

Herr RD, Zun L, Matthews JJ (1989) A directed approach to the dizzy patient. Annals of Emergency Medicine 18, 664–672.

Highstein SM (1991) The central nervous system efferent control of the organs of balance and equilibrium. Neuroscience Research 12, 13–30.

Highstein SM, Goldberg JM, Moschovakis AK, Fernandez C (1987) Inputs from regularly and irregularly discharging vestibular nerve afferents to secondary neurons in the vestibular nuclei of the squirrel monkey. II Correlation with output pathways of secondary neurons. Journal of Neurophysiology 58, 719–738.

HMSO (1992) The Health of the Nation: A Strategy for Health in England. London: HMSO.

Hood JD (1973) Persistence of response in the caloric test. Aerospace Medicine 44, 444–449.

Hood J (1984a) The electro-nystagmographic investigation of spontaneous nystagmus and other disorders of eye movement. In: M Dix, J Hood (eds). Vertigo. Chichester: John Wiley & Sons, pp. 91–112.

Hood J (1984b) Tests of vestibular function. In: M Dix, J Hood (eds). Vertigo. Chichester: John Wiley & Sons, pp. 55–89.

Horak FB (1994) Balance rehabilitation for vestibular and central neural lesions. In: K Taguchi, M Igareshi, S Mori (eds). Vestibular and Neural Front. London: Elsevier Science, pp. 205–213.

Horak FB, Shupert CL (1994) Role of the vestibular system in postural control. In: S Herdman (ed.). Vestibular Rehabilitation. Philadelphia: FA Davis, pp. 22–42.

Horak FB, Shupert CL, Mirka A (1989) Components of postural dyscontrol in the elderly: a review. Neurobiology of Ageing 10, 727–728.

Howton K, Salkovskis PM, Kirk J, Clark DM (1990) Cognitive Behaviour Therapy for Psychiatric Problems – A Practical Guide. Oxford: Oxford Medical Publications.

Hudspeth AJ, Corey DP (1977) Sensitivity, polarity, and conductance change in the response of vertebrate hair cells to controlled mechanical stimuli. Proceedings of the National Academy of Sciences USA 74, 2407–2411.

Igarashi M, Levy JK, Ouchi T, Reschke MF (1981) Further study of physical exercise and locomotor balance compensation after unilateral labyrinthectomy in squirrel monkeys. Acta Otolaryngologica 92, 101–105.

Ito M (1972). Neural design of the cerebellar motor control system. Brain Research 40, 81–84.

Ito M (1975) The vestibulo-cerebellar relationship: vestibulo-ocular reflex arc and flocculus. In: R Nauton (ed.). The Vestibular System. New York: Academic Press, pp. 129–146.

Jacobson GP, Newman CW (1990) The development of the dizziness handicap inventory. Archives of Otolaryngology, Head and Neck Surgery 116, 424–427.

Jensen DE (1979) Reflex control of acute postural asymmetry and compensatory symmetry after a unilateral vestibular lesion. Neurosciences 4, 1059–1073.

Johnson P, Manchester J, Sugden J (1985) Anxiety. Nursing 34, 1008–1012.

de Jong PIVM, de Jong JMVB, Cohen B, Jongkees LBW (1977) Ataxia and nystagmus induced by injection of local anaesthetic in the neck. Annals of Neurology 1, 240–246.

Jongkees LBW, Maas JPM, Philipzoon AJ (1962) Clinical nystagmography. Practica Otolaryngologica 24, 65–89.

Kasai T, Zee DS (1978) Eye-head coordination in labyrinthine-defective human beings. Brain Research 144, 123–141.

Kayan A (1987) Diagnostic tests of balance. In: S Stephens (ed.). Scott Brown's Otolaryngology (fifth edition) Volume 2. London: Butterworths, pp. 304–367.

Keable D (1989) The Management of Anxiety: A Manual for Therapists. London: Churchill-Livingstone.

Keshner EA (1994) Mechanisms controlling posture and balance. Physical Therapy Practice 3, 207–217.

Kety SS, Schmidt CF (1948) The effects of altered arterial tensions of carbon dioxide and oxygen on cerebral blood flow and cerebral oxygen consumption on normal young men. Journal of Clinical Investigation 27, 484–492.

Kikuchi T, Takasaka T, Tonosaki A, Watanabe H (1989) Fine structure of guinea-pig vestibular kinocilium. Acta Otolaryngologica 108, 26–30.

Kileny P (1985) Evaluation of vestibular function. In: J Katz (ed.). Handbook of Clinical Audiology. Baltimore, MD: Williams & Wilkins, pp. 582–603.

Kimura RS (1969) Distribution, structure and function of dark cells in the vestibular labyrinth. Annals of Otology, Rhinology and Laryngology 78, 542–561.

Kirk C, Saunders M (1977) Primary psychiatric illness in a neurological outpatient department in north-east England. Journal of Psychosomatic Research 21, 1–5.

Krebs DE, Gill-Body KM, Ripley PO, Parker SW (1993) Double-blind, placebo-controlled trial of rehabilitation for bilateral vestibular rehabilitation: preliminary report. Otolaryngology, Head and Neck Surgery 109, 735–741.

Kroenke K, Lucas CA, Rosenberg ML, Scherokman B, Herbers JE, Wehrle PA, Boggi JO (1992) Causes of persistent dizziness. Annals of International Medicine 117, 898–904.

Lacour M (1989) Vestibular Compensation: Facts, Theories and Clinical Perspectives. Amsterdam: Elsevier.

Lacour M, Xerri C (1984) Vestibular compensation: new perspectives. In Flohr H, Precht W (eds). Lesion-induced Neuronal Plasticity in Sensorimotor Systems. Berlin: Springer-Verlag, pp. 240–253.

Lacour M, Roll JP, Appaix M (1976) Modifications and development of spinal reflexes in the adult baboon (Papio papio) following unilateral vestibular neurotomy. Brain Research 113, 255–269.

Lang P (1971) The application of psychophysiological methods to the study of psychotherapy and behaviour modification. In: AE Bergin, SL Garfield (eds). Handbook of Psychotherapy and Behaviour Change. New York: Wiley, pp. 75–125

Leigh RG (1994) Pharmacological and optical methods of treating vestibular disorders and nystagmus. In: S Herdman (ed.). Vestibular Rehabilitation. Philadelphia: FA Davis, pp. 185–192.

Leigh RG, Zee DS (1991) The Neurology of Eye Movements. Philadelphia: FA Davis.

Lewis BI (1954) Chronic hyperventilation syndrome. Journal of the American Medical Association 155, 1204–1208.

Lerner Washko N, Gilbert J (1991) Balance retraining: a comprehensive approach to treatment of patients with dizziness and imbalance. Seminars in Hearing 12, 279–295.

Lim DJ (1984) The development and structure of otoconia. In: I Friedman, J Ballantyne (eds). Ultrastructural Atlas of the Inner Ear. London: Butterworth, pp. 245–269.

Lopez I, Meza G (1988) Neurochemical evidence for afferent GABAergic and efferent cholinergic neurotransmission in the frog vestibule. Neuroscience 25, 13–18.

Ludman H (1984) Surgical treatment of vertigo. In: MR Dix, JD Hood (eds). Vertigo. Chichester: John Wiley, pp. 113–132.

Lum LC (1976) The syndrome of chronic habitual hyperventilation. In: OW Hill (ed.). Modern Trends in Psychosomatic Medicine. London: Butterworth, pp. 196–230.

Luxon LM (1996) Post-traumatic vertigo. In: RW Baloh, M Halmagyi (eds). Handbook of Neuro-otology/Vestibular System. New York: Oxford University Press, 381–395.

McCabe BF, Ryu JH, Sekitani T (1972) Further experiments on vestibular compensation. Laryngoscope 82, 381–397.

McCloskey DJ (1978) Kinesthetic sensibility. Physiological Reviews 58, 763–820.

McLaren JW, Hillman DE (1979) Displacement of the semicircular cupula during sinusoidal rotation. Neurosciences Abstracts 3, 544 Abstract 1730.

Mace CJ, Trimble MR (1991) 'Hysteria', 'functional' or 'psychogenic'? A survey of British neurologists' preferences. Journal of the Royal Society of Medicine 84, 471–475.

Magarian GJ (1982) Hyperventilation syndromes: infrequently recognised common expressions of anxiety and stress. Medicine 61, 219–236.

Marks IM (1975) Behavioural treatment of phobic and obsessive-compulsive disorders: a cortical appraisal. Progress In Behaviour Modification 1, 66–158.

Marks IM (1978) Living with Fear. Understanding and Coping with Anxiety. New York: McGraw-Hill.

Marks IM (1981) Space 'phobia': a pseudo-agoraphobic syndrome. Journal of Neurology, Neurosurgery and Psychiatry 44, 387–391.

Marks IM (1987) Fears, Phobias and Rituals. Oxford: Oxford University Press.

Marks IM, Lader M (1973) Anxiety states (anxiety neurosis): a review. Journal of Nervous and Mental Disease 156, 3–18.

Markham CH, Yagi T, Curthoys IS (1977) The contribution of the contralateral labyrinth to second order vestibular neuronal activity in the cat. Brain Research 138, 99–109.

Massion J (1994) Postural control system. Current Opinion in Neurobiology 4, 877–887.

Mathog RH, Peppard SB (1982) Exercise and recovery from vestibular injury. American Journal of Otolaryngology 3, 397–407.

Melvill Jones G (1974) The functional significance of semicircular size. In: HH Kornhuber (ed). Basic Mechanisms. Volume VI Vestibular System (Part 1) Handbook of Sensory Physiology. Berlin: Springer-Verlag, pp. 171–184.

Merchant SN, Rauch SD, Nadol JB (1995) Ménière's disease. European Archives of Otorhinolaryngology 252, 63–75.

Metcalfe T, Gresty MA (1991) Self-controlled reorienting movements in response to rotational displacements in normal subjects and patients with labyrinthine disease. In: B Cohen, DL Yomko, F Guedry (eds). Sensing and Controlling Motion: Proceedings of the New York Academy of Sciences 656, 695–698.

Miller NE (1969) Learning of visceral and glandular responses. Science 163, 434–445.

Millikan CM, Siekert RD (1955) The syndrome of intermittent insufficiency of the basilar arterial system. Mayo Clinic Proceedings 30, 61–68.

Mitchell L (1977) Simple Physiological Relaxation. London: John Murray.

Mitchelson L, Ascher L (1986) Anxiety and Stress Disorders: Cognitive Behavioural Assessment and Treatment. New York: Guilford Press.

Nakagawa H, Ohashi N, Kanda K, Watanabe Y (1993) Autonomic nervous system disturbances as etiological background of vertigo and dizziness. Acta Otolaryngologica Supplementum 504, 130–133.

Nedzelski JM, Barber HO, McIlmoyl L (1986) Diagnoses in a dizziness unit. Journal of Otolaryngology 15, 101–104.

Norré ME (1984) Treatment of unilateral vestibular hypofunction. In: WJ Oosterveld (ed.). Otoneurology. New York: John Wiley, pp. 23–39.

Norré ME (1987) Rationalle of rehabilitation treatment for vertigo. American Journal of Otolaryngology 8, 31–35.

Norré ME (1993) Sensory interaction testing in platform posturography. Journal of Laryngology and Otology 107, 496–501.

Norré ME (1994) Vestibular patients examined by posturography: sensory interaction testing. Journal of Otolaryngology 23, 399–405.

Norré ME, Beckers A (1987) Exercise treatment for paroxysmal positional vertigo: comparison of two types of exercises. Archives of Otorhinolaryngology 244, 291–294.

Norré ME, Beckers A (1988) Comparative study of two types of exercise treatment for paroxysmal positional nystagmus. Annals of Otorhinolaryngology 93, 595–599.

Norré ME, De Weerdt W (1980a) Treatment of vertigo based upon habituation. I. Physiopathological basis. Journal of Laryngology and Rhinology 94, 689–696.

Norré ME, De Weerdt W (1980b) Treatment of vertigo based upon habituation. II. Technique and results of habituation training. Journal of Laryngology and Rhinology 94, 971–977.

Norré ME, De Weerdt W (1981) Positional (provoked) vertigo treated by postural training. Aggressologie 22, 37.

Norré ME, Forrez G, Beckers A (1987) Vestibular dysfunction causing instability in aged patients. Acta Otolaryngologica 104, 50–55.

Noyes R, Clancy J (1976) Anxiety neurosis: a five-year follow-up. Journal of Nervous and Mental Disease 162, 200–205.

Noyes R, Clancy J, Hoenk PR, Slymen DJ (1980) The prognosis of anxiety neurosis. Archives of General Psychiatry 37, 173–178.

O'Leary DP, Davis LL (1990) High frequency autorotational testing of the vestibulo-ocular reflex. Neurologic Clinics 8, 297–312.

O'Leary DP, Davis LL (1994) Vestibular autorotation with active head movements. In: RK Jackler, DE Brackman (eds). Neurotology. St Louis, MI: Mosley, pp. 229–240.

O'Leary DP, Davis LL, Suann LI (1995) Predictive monitoring of high frequency vestibulo-ocular reflex rehabilitation following gentamicin toxicity. Acta Otolaryngologica Supplementum 520, 202–204.

O'Mahoney C, Luxon LM (1996) Causes of balance disorders. In: Chapter 20, AG Kerr (ed.). Scott–Brown's Otolaryngology 2. London: Butterworths, pp. 1–58.

Page NGR, Gresty MA (1985) Motorists' vestibular disorientation syndrome. Journal of Neurology, Neurosurgery and Psychology 48, 729–735.

Parnes LS, McClure JA (1991) Posterior semicircular canal occlusion in the normal ear. Otolaryngology, Head and Neck Surgery 104, 52–57.

de Paulo JR, Folstein MF (1978) Psychiatric disturbance in neurological patients: detection, recognition and hospital course. Annals of Neurology 4, 225–228.

Petrone D, de Benedittis G, de Candia N (1991) Experimental research on vestibular compensation using posturography. Bollettino — Societa Italiana Biologia Sperimentale 67, 731–737.

Pitts FN (1969) The biochemistry of anxiety. Scientific American 220, 69–75.

Pompeiano O (1974) Cerebello–vestibular interactions. In: HH Kornhuber (ed.). Basic Mechanisms Volume VI Vestibular System (Part 1) Handbook of Sensory Physiology. Berlin: Springer-Verlag, pp. 417–476.

Pompeiano O (1994) Neural mechanisms of postural control. In: K Taguchi, M Igarashi, S Mori (eds). Vestibular and Neural Front. London: Elsevier Science, pp. 423–436.

Precht W, Shimazu H, Markham CH (1966) A mechanism of central compensation of vestibular function following hemilabyrinthectomy. Journal of Neurophysiology 29, 996–1010.

Rachman SJ (1977) The conditioning theory of fear-acquisition: a critical examination. Behavioural Research and Therapy 15, 375–387.

Rachman SJ, Hodgson R (1974) Synchrony and desynchrony in fear and avoidance. Behaviour Research and Therapy 12, 311–318.

Raichle ME, Posner JB, Plum F (1970) Cerebral blood flow during and after hyperventilation. Archives of Neurology 23, 394–403.

Raphan T, Matsuo V, Cohen B (1979) Velocity storage in the vestibulo-ocular reflex arc (VOR). Experimental Brain Research 35, 229–248.

Research and Development Task Force (1994). Supporting Research and Development in the NHS (Culyer Report). London: HMSO.

Richmond FJR, Bakker DA (1982) Anatomical organisation and sensory receptor content of soft tissues surrounding upper cervical vertebrae in the cat. Journal of Neurophysiology 48, 49–61.

Roberts TDM (1978) Neurophysiology of Postural Mechanisms (second edition). London: Butterworths.

Rosenberg W, Donald A (1995) Evidence-based medicine: an approach to clinical problem solving. British Medical Journal 310, 1122–1126.

Roucoux A (1992) Eye–head coordination. In: GE Stelmach, J Requin (eds). Tutorials in Motor Behaviour. London: Elsevier Science, pp. 901–917.

Roydhouse N (1974) Vertigo and its treatment. Drugs 7, 297–309.

Rudge P, Chambers BR (1982) Physiological basis for enduring vestibular symptoms. Journal of Neurology, Neurosurgery and Psychiatry 45, 126–130.

Sartory G (1983) Benzodiazepines and behavioural treatment of phobic anxiety. Behavioural Psychiatry 11, 204–217.

Savundra PA, Breckenreg J, Sutherland R, Carter J, Coelho A, Davies RA, Mossman S, Luxon LM (1993) A comparison of the Cawthorne Cooksey exercises and relaxation therapy in the management of vertigo due to peripheral vestibular pathology. 7th International Symposium on Audiological Medicine. Cardiff: Fingerprints, p. 98.

Savundra PA, Luxon LM (1997) The physiology of vertigo and its application to the dizzy patient. In: A Kerr (ed.). Volume I. Scott–Brown's Otolaryngology. London: Butterworths.

Schaefer KP, Meyer DL (1973) Compensatory mechanisms following labyrinthine lesions in the guinea-pig. A simple model of learning. In: HP Zippel (ed.). Memory and Transfer of Information. New York: Plenum, pp. 203–232.

Schaefer KP, Meyer DL (1981) Aspects of vestibular compensation in guinea-pigs. In: H Flohr, W Precht (eds). Lesion-induced Neuronal Plasticity in Sensorimotor Systems. Amsterdam: Springer-Verlag, pp. 197–207.

Schuknecht H (1969) Cupulolithiasis. Archives of Otolaryngology 90, 765–778.

Schuknecht H, Ruby R (1973) Cupulolithiasis. Advances in Otorhinolaryngology 20, 343–443.

Semont A, Freyss G, Vitte E (1988) Curing the BPPV with a liberatory manoeuvre. Advances in Otorhinolaryngology 42, 290–293.

Shepard NT, Telian SA (1995) Programmatic vestibular rehabilitation. Otolaryngology, Head and Neck Surgery 112, 173–181.

Shepard NT, Telian SA, Smith-Wheelock M (1990) Habituation and balance training therapy. Neurologic Clinics 8, 459–475.

Shepard NT, Raj A, Telian SA, Smith-Wheelock M, Anil R (1993) Vestibular and balance rehabilitation therapy. Annals of Otology, Rhinology and Laryngology 102, 198–204.

Shimazu M, Precht W (1966) Inhibition of central vestibular neurons from the contralateral labyrinth and its mediating pathway. Journal of Neurophysiology 29, 467–492.

Shumway-Cook A, Horak FB (1986) Assessing the influence of sensory interaction on balance: suggestions from the field. Physical Therapy 66, 1548–1550.

Shumway-Cook A, Horak FB (1989) Vestibular rehabilitation: an exercise approach to managing symptoms of vestibular dysfunction. Seminars in Hearing 10, 196–207.

Shumway-Cook A, Horak FB (1990) Rehabilitation strategies for patients with vestibular deficits. Neurology Clinics of North America 8, 441–457.

Shumway-Cook A, Woollacott M (1995a) Control of posture and balance. In: A Shumway-Cook, M Woollacott (eds). Motor Control: Theory and Practical Applications. London: Williams & Wilkins, pp. 119–143.

Shumway-Cook A, Woollacott M (1995b) Assessment and treatment of patients with postural disorders. In: A Shumway-Cook, M Woollacott (eds). Motor Control: Theory and Practical Applications. London: Williams & Wilkins, pp. 207–339.

Shumway-Cook A, Woollacott M (1995c) Assessment and treatment of patients with upper extremity manipulatory dyscontrol. In: A Shumway-Cook, M Woollacott (eds). Motor Control: Theory and Practical Applications. London: Williams & Wilkins, pp. 417–447.

Shumway-Cook A, Horak FB, Yardley A, Bronstein AM (1996) Rehabilitation of balance disorders in the patient with vestibular pathology. In: AM Bronstein, T Brandt, M Woollacott (eds). Clinical Disorders of Balance, Posture and Gait. London: Arnold, pp. 211–236.

Shupert CL, Horak FB, Black FO (1994) Hip sway associated with vestibulopathy. Journal of Vestibular Research 4, 231–244.

Shy GM, Drager GA (1960) A neurological syndrome associated with orthostatic hypotension. Archives of Neurology Chicargo 2, 511.

Silver BV, Blanchard EB (1978) Biofeedback and relaxation training in the treatment of psychophysiological disorders: or are the machines really necessary? Cited in D Keable (1989) The Management of Anxiety: A Manual for Therapists. London: Churchill-Livingstone, p. 98.

Singerman (1980) Emotional disturbance in hearing clinic patients. British Journal of Psychiatry 137, 58–62.

Sloane PD, Hartman M, Mitchell CM (1994) Psychological factors associated with chronic dizziness in patients aged 60 and older. Journal of American Geriatric Society 42, 847–852.

Smith DB (1990) Dizziness: a clinical perspective. Neurologic Clinics 8, 199–207.

Smith PF, Curthoys IS (1988) Neuronal activity in the ipsilateral medial vestibular nucleus of the guinea-pig following unilateral labyrinthectomy. Brain Research 444, 308–319.

Smith PF, Curthoys IS (1989) Mechanisms of recovery following unilateral labyrinthectomy: a review. Brain Research Reviews 14, 155–180.

Smith PF, Darlington CL (1991) Neurochemical mechanisms of recovery from peripheral vestibular lesions (vestibular compensation). Brain Research Reviews 16, 117–133.

Smith-Wheelock, Shepard NT, Telian SA (1991) Long-term effects for treatment of balance dysfunction: utilising a home exercise approach. Seminars in Hearing 12, 297–302.

Soley MH, Shock NW (1938) The aetiology of effort syndrome. American Journal of Medical Science 196, 840–851.

Steinhausen W (1931) Über den Nachweis der Bewegung der Cupula in der intakten Bogengangsampulle des Labyrinthes bei der natürlichen rotatorishen und calorishen Reizung. Pflugers Archiv für die gesamte Physiologie des Menschen und der Tiere 228, 322–328.

Stephens SDG, Hogan S, Meredith R (1991) The desynchrony between complaints and signs of vestibular disorders. Acta Otolaryngologica 3 (Supplementum 476) 77–85.

Sterman MB (1974) Neurophysiological and clinical studies of sensorimotor EEG biofeedback training. Some effects on epilepsy. Cited in Health Media & Education Centre (1987) Teaching People to Unwind: Relaxation and Stress Management Techniques. Department of New South Wales: State Health Publication No. (HMEC) 87-022, p. 53.

Stern R, Marks IM (1973) Brief and prolonged flooding. Archives of General Psychiatry 29, 270–276.

Takahashi M, Hoshikawa H, Tsujita N, Akiyama I (1988) Effect of labyrinthine dysfunction upon head ossilation during stepping and running. Acta Otolaryngologica 106, 348–353.

Takemori S, Ida M, Umezu H (1985) Vestibular training after sudden loss of vestibular functions. Otology, Rhinology and Laryngology 47, 76–83.

Tanaka M, Takeda N, Senba E, Tohyama M, Kubo T, Matsunga T (1989) Localisation, origin and fine structure of calcistonin gene related peptide containing fibres in vestibular end organs of the rat. Brain Research 504, 31–35.

Theunissen EJJM, Huygen PLM, Folering HT (1986) Vestibular hyperreactivity and hyperventilation. Cited in L Yardley (1994) Vertigo and Dizziness. London: Routledge, p. 80.

Tyler P, Murphy S (1987) The place of benzodiazepines in psychiatric practice. British Journal of Psychiatry 151, 719–723.

Usami S, Hozawa J, Ylikoski J (1991) Co-existence of Substance P and calcitonin gene related peptide like immunoreactivity in rat vestibular end organs. Acta Otolaryngologica Supplementum 481, 168–169.

Vercher JL, Magenes G, Preblanc C, Gauthier GM (1994) Eye–head–hand coordination in pointing at visual targets: spatial and temporal analysis. Experimental Brain Research 99, 507–523.

Wersall J, Bagger-Sjoback D (1974) Morphology of the vestibular sense organs. In: HH Kornhuber (ed.). Basic Mechanisms. Volume VI. Vestibular System (Part 1) Handbook of Sensory Physiology. Berlin: Springer-Verlag, pp. 123–170.

Wist ER, Brandt T, Krafczyk S (1983) Oscillopsia and retinal slip. Brain 106, 153–168.

World Health Organization (1980) International Classification of Impairments, Disabilities and Handicaps. Geneva: WHO.

World Health Organization (1988) The clinical investigation of drugs for the treatment of involuntary movement disorders. Clinical Consensus Documents 9. Copenhagen: WHO.

Yardley L (1994) Vertigo and Dizziness. London: Routledge.

Yardley L, Putman J (1992) Quantitative analysis of factors contributing to handicap and distress in vertiginous patients: a questionnaire study. Clinical Otolaryngology 17, 231–236.

Yardley L, Luxon LM (1994) Treating dizziness with vestibular rehabilitation. British Medical Journal 308, 1252–1253.

Yardley L, Masson E, Verschuur C, Haacke N, Luxon LM (1992) Symptoms, anxiety and handicap in dizzy patients: development of the vertigo symptom scale. Journal of Psychosomatic Research 36, 731–741.

Yee RD, Baloh RW, Honrubia V, Jenkins HA (1982) Pathophysiology of optokinetic nystagmus. In: V Honrubia, M Brazier (eds). Nystagmus and Vertigo: Clinical Approaches to the Patient with Dizziness. New York: Academic Press, pp. 251–275.

Zee D (1988) The management of patients with vestibular disorders. In: HO Barber, JA Sharpe (eds). Vestibular Disorders. Chicago, IL: Year Book Medical Publishers, pp. 254–274.

Zee DS, Yee RD, Robinson DA (1976) Optokinetic responses in labyrinthine defective human beings. Brain Research 113, 423–428.

# Index